MW00947381

The Ultimate Lean & Green Cookbook for Beginners

Master 1800 Days of Fueling Hacks & Nutritious Green Recipes. Embark on a Weight Loss Journey, Reinvent Your Health & Physique with a 30-day Meal Plan.

Tessa Maddox

Table of Contents

Introduction

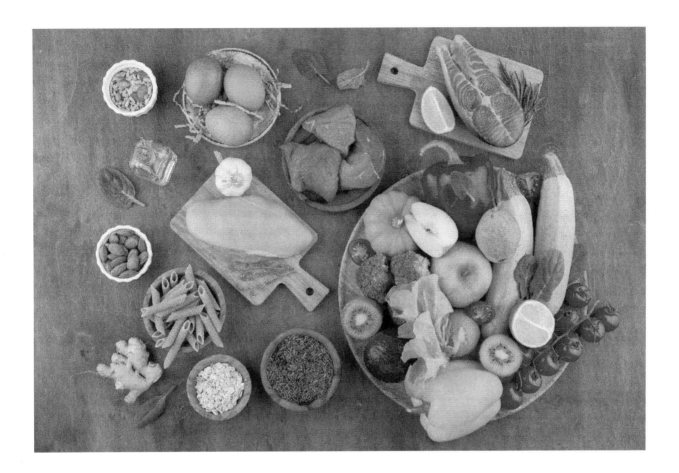

Welcome to a Healthier You

Welcome to a world where health and flavor harmoniously blend, creating a symphony of taste and nourishment. You're about to embark on a culinary journey that redefines the relationship between the body, mind, and plate. This journey is about embracing a lifestyle that balances taste, health, and sustainability.

The Lean and Green Philosophy

At the heart of our journey is the Lean and Green philosophy—a way of life that celebrates the power of plant-based foods. These foods are not just fuel for the body; they are an expression of our connection to nature and a commitment to our health. This book is a gateway to explore the richness of plant-based eating, offering a collection of recipes and insights to ignite your passion for wholesome, natural foods.

Whether you're a committed vegan, exploring vegetarianism, or simply looking to integrate more plant-based meals into your diet, this book caters to you. It's designed to be inclusive, offering a range of recipes and tips that appeal to various tastes and dietary needs. Our goal is to make plant-based eating accessible, enjoyable, and deeply satisfying.

Beyond Just Eating

This journey goes beyond the act of eating. It's about understanding the impact of food choices on our health and the environment. It's a path to discovering how nourishing your body with plant-based foods can be an enriching, life-changing experience.

As you turn each page, let yourself be inspired by the potential that lies in every ingredient, every meal, every bite. We encourage you to embrace this journey with an open heart and a curious palate. Let this book be a companion as you explore the myriad possibilities of plant-based cooking and the joy it brings.

Welcome to a journey that's not just about eating, but about living. Welcome to a Healthier You.

The Power of Lean and Green

The Power of Lean and Green is not just a dietary choice; it's a revolution in how we think about and consume food. This approach intertwines the simplicity of lean proteins and the richness of green, plant-based foods, creating a synergy that revitalizes our eating habits. It's a testament to how we can thrive on meals that are both nourishing and environmentally conscious.

The Core Philosophy

At its core, Lean and Green is about balance and harmony. It's a culinary philosophy that promotes a diet rich in vegetables, fruits, lean proteins, and whole grains. This way of eating is not just about reducing calories or cutting out food groups; it's about enriching your diet with a diverse range of nutrients that support your body's natural health and well-being. Lean and Green goes beyond personal health, advocating for a sustainable approach to eating. By emphasizing plant-based ingredients, this diet contributes to a smaller carbon footprint and a more sustainable agricultural system. It's about making choices that are good for you and the planet, striking a balance between ecological responsibility and nutritional richness.

Adaptable and Inclusive

One of the most beautiful aspects of the Lean and Green approach is its adaptability. Whether you're a meat-eater looking to incorporate more plant-based meals into your diet, a vegetarian, or a vegan, this approach offers flexibility and inclusivity.

It celebrates the diversity of diets and encourages a tailored approach to meet individual dietary needs and preferences.

A Path to Enhanced Well-being

Embracing Lean and Green is more than a diet; it's a path to enhanced well-being. It's about discovering the joy of cooking with whole, unprocessed foods and experiencing the burst of energy and vitality that comes from nourishing your body with the best nature has to offer. It's about feeling good, inside and out, knowing that your food choices are contributing to a healthier self and a healthier world.

As you delve into this book, you'll uncover the secrets of Lean and Green—how it revitalizes your body, transforms your cooking, and brings a new, vibrant perspective to your plate. Get ready to embark on a journey that will not only change the way you eat but also the way you perceive and interact with food. Welcome to the transformative Power of Lean and Green.

Understanding the Fundamentals

At its core, the Lean and Green approach transcends the traditional diet mindset. It's a commitment to a sustainable lifestyle that harmonizes body wellness with environmental respect. Here, we explore the basic principles that form the bedrock of this philosophy, focusing not just on weight loss but on a profound, enduring transformation in how we relate to food and health.

Nutritional Balance and Sustainability

Central to Lean and Green is the nutritional synergy between lean proteins and green, plant-based foods. This union delivers a nutrient-rich diet, brimming with essential amino acids, vitamins, minerals, and fiber. We delve into how this synergy not only satiates but also energizes and revitalizes.

Moreover, we emphasize sustainability, advocating for environmentally conscious food choices like locally sourced and organic produce. This approach isn't just about personal health; it's about nurturing our planet.

Lean and Green stands out for its adaptability. Whether you're vegetarian, vegan, or have specific dietary needs, this approach molds to fit your lifestyle, ensuring inclusivity at its heart. Beyond diet, Lean and Green embodies a holistic view of health, intertwining mindful eating, physical activity, adequate rest, and stress management. This chapter sets the stage for a transformative journey, guiding you towards a healthier, more balanced life with Lean and Green.

Chapter 1: Starting with the Basics

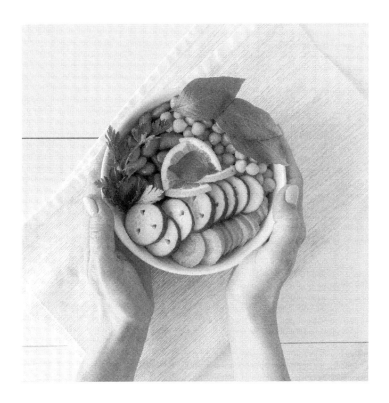

What is the Lean and Green Diet?

The Lean and Green Diet isn't just a diet; it's a lifestyle choice, intertwining the wisdom of nutrition science with the essence of environmental sustainability.

At its heart, it combines lean proteins – from both animal and plant sources – with a plethora of green, leafy vegetables and other plant-based foods.

This fusion creates a harmonious balance of macronutrients, ensuring your body gets the right mix of proteins, healthy fats, and complex carbohydrates, all while emphasizing low-calorie, high-nutrient options.

Customizability for Diverse Lifestyles

What sets the Lean and Green Diet apart is its adaptability to various dietary preferences and restrictions. Whether you're a meat-lover, vegetarian, or vegan, this diet molds to meet your nutritional needs. It's designed to be inclusive, acknowledging the diverse food choices and lifestyle requirements of individuals. By providing a template rather than strict rules, it offers flexibility, making healthy eating accessible and enjoyable for everyone.

Focus on Whole, Unprocessed Foods

The Lean and Green Diet encourages a shift from processed foods to whole, unprocessed, and fresh foods. This means embracing fruits, vegetables, whole grains, and lean proteins in their most natural form. The diet advocates for cooking methods that preserve the nutritional integrity of foods, such as steaming, grilling, and sautéing, steering clear of unhealthy fats and excess sugars. This approach not only nourishes the body but also respects the environment, promoting sustainable eating habits.

Through these guiding principles, the Lean and Green Diet emerges as more than just a pathway to weight loss or health maintenance. It represents a holistic approach to eating and living, where food choices reflect a deeper understanding of nutrition and environmental stewardship.

The Science Behind the Meals

The Lean and Green Diet is more than a set of meal suggestions; it's a scientifically-crafted approach to eating. It leverages the synergy between lean proteins and green, fiber-rich vegetables, creating a diet that balances essential nutrients effectively. This synergy ensures that each meal delivers a balanced array of macronutrients – proteins for muscle repair and growth, carbohydrates for energy, and fats for cellular health – while also providing a rich supply of vitamins and minerals.

Impact on Metabolism and Health

The diet's structure is designed to stabilize blood sugar levels, reducing the spikes and crashes often associated with processed food consumption. The inclusion of ample greens and vegetables ensures a high intake of dietary fiber, which aids in digestive health and satiety. This combination of protein and fiber has a positive impact on metabolism, aiding in weight management and reducing the risk of chronic diseases such as Type 2 diabetes and heart disease.

Psychological Benefits

From a psychological standpoint, the Lean and Green Diet doesn't just focus on what you eat, but how you eat. Mindful eating practices are encouraged, promoting a deeper connection with food and its impact on the body. This approach helps in developing a healthier relationship with food, viewing it as a source of nourishment and energy rather than just a means of quelling hunger or satisfying cravings.

In summary, the Lean and Green Diet's effectiveness lies in its evidence-based approach, combining the right foods in the right proportions to maximize health benefits. It's a holistic diet plan that considers not just the physical, but also the psychological aspects of eating, providing a comprehensive pathway to a healthier lifestyle.

Benefits of Going Lean and Green

1. Enhanced Nutritional Balance: The Lean and Green diet is more than a meal plan; it's a balanced approach to eating. By focusing on lean proteins and a variety of green vegetables, this diet ensures an optimal balance of essential nutrients. Proteins support muscle and tissue health, while green vegetables provide a rich source of vitamins, minerals, and fiber. This balance is crucial for maintaining bodily functions and overall health.

2. Weight Management and Metabolic Health: One of the most significant benefits of this diet is its impact on weight management. The high protein content increases satiety, reducing the urge for frequent snacking or overeating. Moreover, lean proteins and greens have a positive effect on metabolism, aiding in weight loss and maintenance. By stabilizing blood sugar levels, this diet also plays a crucial role in preventing and managing diabetes.

3. Heart Health and Reduced Disease Risk: A diet rich in vegetables and lean proteins has been linked to a reduced risk of heart disease. The Lean and Green diet is low in unhealthy fats and high in fiber, which helps lower cholesterol levels and improves heart health. Additionally, the antioxidants present in green vegetables reduce inflammation, further protecting against chronic diseases.

4. Enhanced Digestive Health: The high fiber content in the Lean and Green diet aids in digestion and promotes gut health. Fiber acts as a prebiotic, feeding beneficial gut bacteria, which is essential for a healthy digestive system. Regular consumption of fiber also helps prevent constipation and other digestive issues.

5. Improved Energy Levels and Mental Clarity: By providing a steady source of energy through balanced meals, the Lean and Green diet enhances overall vitality and mental clarity. Unlike diets high in processed foods and sugars that lead to energy spikes and crashes, this diet ensures a consistent energy supply, helping you stay focused and active throughout the day.

6. Sustainable and Environmentally Friendly: Emphasizing plant-based ingredients, the Lean and Green diet is not only beneficial for health but also for the environment. By reducing the intake of processed foods and focusing on whole, natural ingredients, it promotes sustainable eating habits.

In conclusion, the Lean and Green diet offers a multitude of benefits, from improved physical health and weight management to mental clarity and environmental sustainability. It's a comprehensive approach that goes beyond mere weight loss, fostering a healthier, more balanced lifestyle.

Setting Realistic Expectations

Gradual Changes and Personalization

Embarking on the Lean and Green journey is an adventure in gradual transformation and personal adaptation. It's not about overnight changes but embracing a sustainable shift in lifestyle. Realistic expectations mean recognizing that progress happens over time. This diet isn't a one-size-fits-all solution; it's a canvas for each individual to paint their unique nutritional needs and goals. Whether you're aiming for weight management, improved health, or increased energy levels, the key is to tailor the diet to your personal journey, celebrating small victories along the way.

Balance and Resilience

The Lean and Green lifestyle is more than just dietary changes; it's about embracing balance in all health aspects. A balanced approach integrates not only mindful eating but also regular physical activity, adequate rest, and effective stress management. Understanding that challenges and plateaus are part of this journey is crucial. Mental preparation for these hurdles, whether by leaning on a support community, tweaking your diet, or consulting a professional, forms the backbone of resilience. It's these moments of overcoming obstacles that truly define the success of your journey.

A Lifelong Commitment to Health

Finally, adopting the Lean and Green diet is about a lifelong commitment to health, not just a fleeting goal. It's a continuous process of making healthier choices that seamlessly blend into your daily life. This journey is about a sustainable and enjoyable lifestyle change, not a temporary fix. The focus remains on a long-term dedication to wellness, where the journey itself is as significant as the destination.

In embracing the Lean and Green way of life, you embark on a path of gradual change, balance, and a lasting commitment to your well-being. It's about understanding the journey's nature and being kind to yourself as you navigate this transformative path.

Chapter 2: Ingredients 101

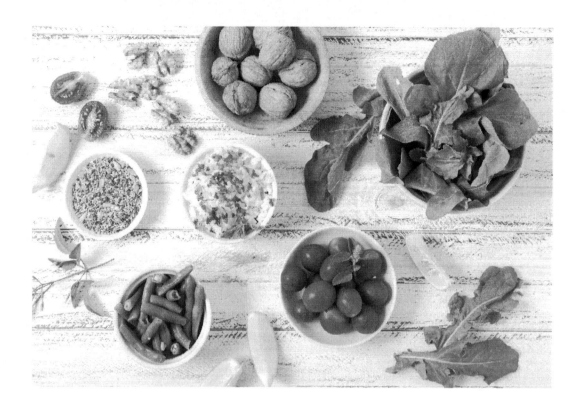

Must-have Pantry Staples

The cornerstone of a Lean and Green kitchen lies in its pantry, filled with whole, unprocessed foods. These staples not only provide the necessary nutrients for a balanced diet but also offer versatility for a range of delicious, healthful meals.

Stocking up on whole grains like quinoa, brown rice, and farro offers a fiber-rich base for meals, ensuring sustained energy levels and digestive health. Legumes, including lentils, chickpeas, and black beans, are indispensable for their protein content and ability to add heartiness to any dish.

Lean Proteins and Healthy Fats

A well-planned pantry caters to both vegetarian and non-vegetarian preferences with a variety of lean protein options. Canned or pouch-packed wild-caught salmon, tuna, and sardines are excellent for quick, protein-packed meals. For plant-based proteins, consider incorporating tofu, tempeh, and a variety of nuts and seeds. Healthy fats are equally important; items like extra-virgin olive oil, avocados, and an assortment of nuts and seeds (such as almonds, chia seeds, and flaxseeds) are essential. These facts are not only crucial for brain health but also help in the absorption of vitamins.

Herbs, Spices, and Flavor Enhancers

The secret to making healthy food delicious lies in the use of herbs and spices. Keeping a diverse range of these can transform any simple dish into a culinary delight. Fresh or dried herbs like basil, thyme, and cilantro, along with spices such as turmeric, cumin, and paprika, are key to adding flavors without extra calories. Natural sweeteners like honey or maple syrup and condiments like low-sodium soy sauce or apple cider vinegar can also provide an extra zing to your meals.

Embracing the Lean and Green lifestyle starts in your pantry. By prioritizing whole foods, lean proteins, healthy fats, and natural flavor enhancers, you set the stage for nutritious and enjoyable meals that align with both your health goals and palate preferences.

Navigating the Fresh Produce Aisle

The Art of Selecting Fresh Produce

Entering the fresh produce aisle can be like stepping into a garden of earthly delights, but knowing how to navigate this space is key. It's not just about colors and textures; it's about understanding freshness and seasonality. Start by focusing on seasonal produce, which guarantees both nutritional density and optimal flavor. A ripe, in-season tomato bursting with juice is not just a culinary pleasure but a nutritional powerhouse. Learn the art of gently pressing for ripeness, observing color vibrancy, and smelling for freshness. These simple acts transform shopping from a mundane task to a sensory adventure.

Organic or Conventional: Making the Choice

The organic versus conventional produce debate is a personal one. Organic produce is grown without synthetic pesticides and fertilizers, offering an eco-friendly option. However, it can be pricier. When budget constraints arise, prioritize organic selections for items known to have higher pesticide residues, like leafy greens and berries. For those with thicker skins or rinds, such as avocados and melons, conventional versions can be a more economical choice without significantly compromising health benefits.

Diversity for Nutritional Balance

The colors in your shopping cart reflect more than just visual appeal; they represent a range of nutrients. Each color in fruits and vegetables is a clue to its nutritional contents – from the beta-carotene in orange carrots to the lycopene in red bell peppers. Aiming for a rainbow assortment ensures a wide range of vitamins, minerals, and antioxidants, catering to all aspects of health, from immune support to anti-inflammatory benefits.

This approach not only enhances your nutrient intake but also adds variety and excitement to your meals.

In conclusion, mastering the fresh produce aisle is an essential skill in the lean and green lifestyle. It's about making informed choices, understanding the nuances of organic versus conventional, and embracing the diversity of nature's bounty. A well-navigated produce aisle leads to a kitchen brimming with possibilities, setting the stage for meals that are as nourishing as they are delightful. Remember, every fruit and vegetable in your basket carries a story – of flavor, nutrition, and the simple joy of eating foods that are in harmony with your body and the planet.

Optimal Protein Choices

In the realm of the Lean and Green diet, the emphasis on plant-based proteins is not just a trend but a healthful pivot. The power of plants in delivering high-quality proteins is often underestimated. Legumes, such as lentils, chickpeas, and black beans, are not only rich in protein but also fiber, which aids in digestion and prolonged satiety. Tofu and tempeh, made from soybeans, stand out as versatile protein sources, effortlessly absorbing flavors and enriching a variety of dishes from stir-fries to salads. Quinoa, a pseudo-cereal, also emerges as a complete protein, providing all nine essential amino acids, which is a rarity in the plant kingdom.

Incorporating Lean Animal Proteins

For those who include animal products in their diet, choosing lean proteins is crucial. Skinless poultry, such as chicken and turkey breast, offer high protein content with minimal saturated fat.

Fish, particularly fatty varieties like salmon and mackerel, are not only lean but also rich in omega-3 fatty acids, beneficial for heart health.

When it comes to red meat, opt for cuts like sirloin or tenderloin and prioritize grass-fed and organic sources to reduce exposure to antibiotics and hormones.

Protein-Rich Dairy Alternatives

Dairy products can be an excellent protein source; however, the Lean and Green lifestyle often calls for low-fat or plant-based alternatives. Greek yogurt, particularly the non-fat variety, is packed with protein and probiotics. In the sphere of plant-based options, almond milk, soy milk, and coconut yogurt are popular choices. They cater to those with lactose intolerance or dairy sensitivities and can be easily incorporated into smoothies, cereals, and baking recipes.

In conclusion, the world of protein within the Lean and Green framework is diverse and adaptable to various dietary preferences and needs. Whether it's through plant-based sources or lean animal proteins, the goal is to fuel the body with high-quality, nutrient-dense options. Protein is not just a macronutrient; it's a vital component of a balanced diet that supports muscle maintenance, energy levels, and overall health. So, as you navigate your protein choices, remember that variety and quality are key to a satisfying and healthful dietary journey.

Healthy Fats: Which to Use and When

In the journey towards a balanced Lean and Green diet, understanding the role of healthy fats is essential. Gone are the days of the low-fat craze; today, we embrace fats for their vital role in nutrient absorption, brain health, and satiety.

However, not all fats are created equal. Monounsaturated and polyunsaturated fats, found in sources like olives, nuts, seeds, and fish, are heart-healthy choices.

These fats, especially omega-3 fatty acids from fish like salmon and mackerel, are crucial for cardiovascular health and cognitive function.

Cooking with the Right Oils

 When it comes to cooking, choosing the right oil can make a significant difference. Extra virgin olive oil, rich in monounsaturated fats, is perfect for salad dressings and low-heat cooking. Its flavor and nutritional profile make it a staple in the Lean and Green kitchen. For higher heat cooking, avocado oil and grapeseed oil offer higher smoke points, ensuring that the fats don't break down into harmful compounds. Coconut oil, while higher in saturated fat, can be used sparingly for its unique flavor and medium-chain triglycerides, known for their energy-boosting properties.

Incorporating Nuts and Seeds

Nuts and seeds are more than just snacks; they are powerhouses of healthy fats and essential nutrients. Almonds, walnuts, chia seeds, and flaxseeds are not only great for heart health but also add texture and flavor to meals.
Sprinkling a handful of these onto salads, yogurts, or breakfast cereals is an effortless way to incorporate healthy fats into your diet. They're also a fantastic source of fiber and protein, making them a triple threat in the world of nutrition.

Embracing Avocados and Olives

Avocados and olives are two fruits that are uniquely high in healthy fats. Avocados, with their creamy texture, are incredibly versatile – perfect in smoothies for added richness, as spreads on whole-grain toasts, or simply as a topping in salads and bowls. Olives, with their distinct flavor, can elevate a simple dish to something extraordinary.
 Both are excellent sources of monounsaturated fats, promoting heart health and offering anti-inflammatory benefits.

In conclusion, integrating healthy fats into your Lean and Green diet is not just about adding flavor and richness to your meals; it's about making smart choices that benefit your heart, brain, and overall health. By choosing the right sources of fats, you can enjoy the myriad benefits they offer while maintaining a balanced and healthful diet. So, next time you're in the kitchen, reach for those avocados, nuts, seeds, and quality oils, knowing you're nourishing your body with the best nature has to offer.

Flavor Boosters: Herbs and Spices

In the realm of lean and green eating, the art of seasoning with herbs and spices becomes your secret weapon. It's not just about adding flavor; it's about transforming simple ingredients into culinary masterpieces while keeping health in check. Herbs and spices are the unsung heroes of the kitchen, offering a plethora of flavors without the added calories, fats, or sodium often found in processed seasonings.

Herbs: Fresh vs. Dried

Understanding the difference between fresh and dried herbs is key. Fresh herbs, like basil, cilantro, and parsley, bring a bright, vibrant flavor to dishes, ideal for salads, dressings, and garnishes. On the other hand, dried herbs, such as oregano, thyme, and rosemary, have a more concentrated, robust flavor, perfect for longer cooking processes where they can slowly release their aromas. A general rule of thumb: use fresh herbs towards the end of cooking and dried herbs in the earlier stages.

Spices: A World of Flavors

Spices open up a world of flavors, from the earthy tones of cumin and turmeric to the warm notes of cinnamon and nutmeg. They are not just flavor enhancers but also packed with health benefits. For example, turmeric is known for its anti-inflammatory properties, and cinnamon for its blood sugar regulating abilities. Creating your own spice blends can be a fun and rewarding process, allowing you to control the flavors and avoid the excess salt often found in store-bought mixes.

Aromatic Combinations

Mastering the art of combining herbs and spices can turn your meals from mundane to extraordinary. Imagine the zesty kick of lemon zest and dill on grilled fish, the rich depth of garlic and rosemary in roasted vegetables, or the exotic allure of curry powder in a lentil stew. These combinations do not just add flavor; they create an experience, making your lean and green meals something to look forward to.

Incorporating herbs and spices into your cooking is not only about tantalizing your taste buds; it's about enhancing the natural flavors of your ingredients, adding nutritional value, and making each meal a celebration of health and taste. As you embark on your lean and green journey, let herbs and spices be your guide, turning each dish into a symphony of flavors that nourish both the body and soul. So, go ahead, experiment with that herb garden or that spice rack – your palate and your health will thank you.

Chapter 3: Meal Planning and Prepping

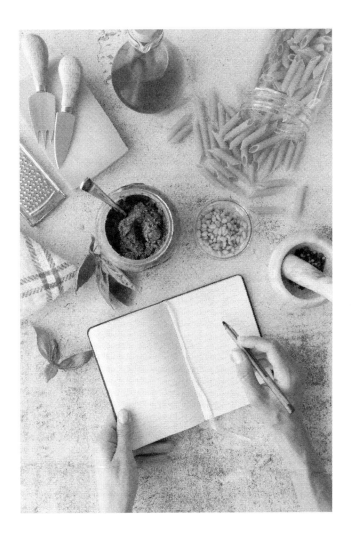

Creating a Weekly Lean and Green Menu

Embarking on a journey of healthy eating begins with a well-thought-out plan. Creating a weekly lean and green menu is not just about listing meals; it's a strategic approach to ensure your diet aligns with your health goals while catering to your taste buds. It's about making smart, delicious choices that are sustainable in the long run.

The Art of Balancing Meals

The core of your weekly menu revolves around balancing macro and micronutrients. Each meal should harmoniously blend proteins, healthy fats, and green vegetables. This not only ensures nutritional adequacy but also keeps your meals interesting. Imagine a plate with grilled salmon (rich in omega-3 fatty acids), a side of sautéed kale (packed with vitamins), and quinoa (a great source of protein and fiber). This approach not only nourishes your body but also keeps your palate engaged.

Theme Your Days for Variety

To avoid monotony, theme your days around different cuisines or meal types. For instance, 'Mediterranean Monday' could feature a vibrant Greek salad, 'Taco Tuesday' could include lean turkey tacos with lettuce wraps, and 'Stir-Fry Friday' could be a celebration of colorful vegetables and tofu in a light soy and ginger sauce. This not only simplifies shopping and preparation but also adds an element of excitement to your weekly eating routine.

Advance Prep: Your Time-Saving Ally

One of the secrets to sticking with a healthy eating plan is preparing in advance. Dedicate a few hours over the weekend to pre-chop vegetables, marinate proteins, and cook grains or legumes. Preparing components of your meals ahead of time makes it easier to assemble healthy dishes quickly during busy weekdays.

Incorporating Flexibility

While structure is important, so is flexibility. Life is unpredictable, and your meal plan should accommodate last-minute changes. Have a few 'emergency' meal ideas that can be quickly put together with pantry staples or freezer ingredients. For instance, a quick bean chili or an omelet loaded with vegetables can be a savior on hectic days.

Mindful Eating: Beyond the Plate

Finally, remember that eating healthily is not just about what's on your plate; it's also about your eating environment and habits. Try to eat mindfully, savoring each bite, and listening to your body's hunger and fullness cues. This holistic approach ensures that your journey to a lean and green lifestyle is enjoyable, sustainable, and beneficial to both body and mind.

In conclusion, creating a weekly lean and green menu is about embracing variety, preparing in advance, and enjoying the process of nourishing your body. It's a blend of science and art - a dance of flavors, nutrients, and textures that come together to form a symphony of wholesome, delicious meals. So, plan, prep, and relish in the joy of eating well.

Portion Control Tips

In the world of lean and green living, understanding and managing portion sizes is crucial. It's about nurturing your body with enough food to energize and heal, without overindulging. This section offers practical tips to help you master portion control, ensuring that each meal is both satisfying and in line with your health goals.

Visual Cues for Portioning: The Art of Estimation

We often eat with our eyes first, and this can be used to our advantage in portion control. Familiarizing yourself with visual cues can make a big difference. For instance, a serving of protein should be the size of your palm, a portion of carbohydrates can be compared to the size of your clenched fist, and a serving of fats should be about the size of your thumb. These simple comparisons are handy tools when you're away from your kitchen scale or measuring cups.

Another effective approach is the plate method. Divide your plate into sections: half of it should be filled with green, non-starchy vegetables, one-quarter with lean protein, and the remaining quarter with whole grains or starchy vegetables. This method ensures a well-balanced meal with appropriate portions of each food group.

Mindful Eating: Tuning into Your Body's Signals

Mindful eating is a crucial aspect of portion control. It involves paying attention to the physical hunger and satiety signals that guide your decisions to start and stop eating. Eating slowly and without distraction allows you to recognize when you are full, reducing the likelihood of overeating.

One of the most effective strategies for portion control is pre-portioning your meals and snacks. This takes the guesswork out of eating and prevents mindless nibbling. By dividing foods into individual servings, you can ensure that each meal or snack you consume is aligned with your dietary goals.

Consistency is Key: Regular Meals and Portions

Establishing a routine can greatly aid in maintaining portion control. Eating at regular intervals prevents extreme hunger that can lead to overeating.

Consistency in your meal schedule and portion sizes helps regulate your body's hunger cues and supports metabolic balance.

Sometimes, it's not just about what you eat, but how you present it. Using smaller plates can trick your brain into feeling more satisfied with a smaller amount of food. It's a simple psychological trick that can lead to significant changes in your eating habits.

In summary, mastering portion control is about more than just measuring food; it's a blend of visual cues, mindful eating, pre-portioning, consistency, and psychological tricks. By incorporating these strategies into your daily routine, you can enjoy a variety of foods while maintaining a balanced diet. Remember, portion control is not about restriction; it's about empowering yourself to eat in a way that nourishes and satisfies your body.

Storage and Freshness Hacks

The key to a successful lean and green diet is not just about selecting the right ingredients; it's also about how you store them to preserve their freshness and nutritional value. This section will delve into effective storage techniques, ensuring that your produce, proteins, and other essentials retain their optimal quality from the store to your plate.

Produce Preservation: Beyond the Fridge

Proper storage of fruits and vegetables can significantly extend their shelf life. Start by understanding which items are best kept at room temperature and which thrive in the cool, humid environment of your refrigerator's crisper drawer.
For example, tomatoes lose flavor in the fridge and are best kept on the countertop, while leafy greens need the moisture of a fridge to stay crisp. Additionally, storing fruits and vegetables separately is essential as some fruits produce ethylene gas, which can prematurely ripen (or spoil) nearby vegetables.

Protein Care: Ensuring Freshness and Safety

Proteins, particularly meats and fish, demand careful handling. To maintain freshness and prevent cross-contamination, store them in the coldest part of your refrigerator or freezer, using airtight containers or wraps. If freezing, consider portioning the protein into individual meal-sized amounts before freezing; this not only saves space but also simplifies meal prep.

Herb Longevity: From Garden to Table

Fresh herbs can elevate any dish, but they often wilt quickly. Extend their life by treating them like a bouquet of flowers: trim the stems and place them in a jar of water, loosely covered with a plastic bag, in the fridge. For heartier herbs like rosemary or thyme, wrapping them in a damp paper towel before refrigerating can keep them fresh for weeks.

Bulk Buys: Organizing Your Pantry

Buying in bulk can be cost-effective, but without proper storage, you risk spoilage. Transfer grains, nuts, seeds, and other dry goods into clear, airtight containers. This not only extends their shelf life but also makes it easy to see what you have at a glance, reducing waste and repeated purchases.

Freezer Finesse: Flash Freezing and Labeling

Make the most of your freezer with flash freezing – a technique where you spread items like berries, sliced vegetables, or meatballs on a tray to freeze individually before transferring them to a container. This prevents clumping and ensures easy portioning. Always label and date your freezer items; not only does this help with inventory management, but it also ensures you use older items first.

Refrigerator Real Estate: Strategic Organization

Organize your refrigerator strategically. Keep ready-to-eat foods and meal preps on the middle and top shelves where they are easily accessible. Store condiments and less perishable items in the door, and reserve the lower shelves for raw ingredients used in cooking.

By implementing these storage and freshness hacks, you're not just preserving food; you're also ensuring that every meal is as nutritious and delicious as possible. These strategies can help reduce food waste, save money, and make your lean and green journey both enjoyable and sustainable. Remember, a well-organized kitchen is the first step to a healthier lifestyle.

Quick and Easy Breakfast Preps

Efficient Morning Solutions with Overnight and Batch Recipes

Beginning your day with a nutritious breakfast is essential, yet often challenging amidst the morning rush. Overnight oats and chia puddings provide a convenient solution.

Simply combine ingredients like rolled oats or chia seeds with almond milk and Greek yogurt in the evening, and wake up to a ready-to-eat, wholesome meal. Additionally, consider batch-baking items like almond butter and banana muffins or spinach and feta mini frittatas during the weekend. These can be stored and conveniently consumed throughout the week, ensuring a healthy start to your busy days.

Freezer-Friendly Breakfasts and Savory Options

Leverage your freezer by preparing and storing breakfast items like whole grain pancakes or waffles. These can be quickly reheated for a speedy morning meal. For those who prefer savory breakfasts, preparing and refrigerating breakfast jars filled with layers of quinoa, avocado, cherry tomatoes, and boiled eggs offers a quick, balanced, and satisfying option. Alternatively, lean turkey or tofu lettuce wraps can be made in advance for a protein-rich start to the day.

Preparation Techniques for Time-Saving Mornings

A little preparation can significantly streamline your morning routine. Assemble smoothie packs with pre-portioned fruits, greens, and protein powder for a quick blend-and-go option. Also, arranging your breakfast ingredients the night before, such as setting out bowls for your overnight oats or prepping your coffee machine, can save valuable time in the morning. These simple yet effective strategies ensure that you don't compromise on a healthy and hearty breakfast, even on the busiest days.

Chapter 4: Lean and Green Breakfast Recipes

Energizing Morning Smoothies

Berry Bliss Smoothie

Preparation time: 5 minutes
Ingredients: 1 cup mixed berries (strawberries, blueberries, raspberries), 1 frozen banana, 1 cup spinach, 1 tablespoon almond butter, 1 teaspoon maca powder, 1½ cups almond milk, 1 scoop plant-based vanilla protein powder
Servings: 2
Mode of cooking: Blend
Procedure: 1. Add all berries, banana, and spinach to blender; 2. Include almond butter and maca powder; 3. Pour in almond milk; 4. Add scoop of protein powder; 5. Blend until creamy.
Nutritional values: Estimated Calories: 320, Protein: 20g, Carbohydrates: 45g, Fat: 8g, Fiber: 9g.

Tropical Green Detox Smoothie

Preparation time: 6 minutes
Ingredients: 1 cup kale leaves, 1 cup tropical mix (pineapple, mango, papaya), ½ avocado, 1 tablespoon chlorella powder, 2 teaspoons fresh ginger, 1½ cups coconut water, 1 tablespoon lemon juice
Servings: 2
Method of cooking: Blend
Procedure: 1. Combine kale and tropical mix in blender; 2. Add avocado and chlorella; 3. Grate ginger into mixture; 4. Pour in coconut water and lemon juice; 5. Blend until smooth.
Nutritional values: Estimated Calories: 235, Protein: 4g, Carbohydrates: 36g, Fat: 10g, Fiber: 7g.

Chocolate Almond Protein Smoothie

Preparation time: 7 minutes
Ingredients: 2 tablespoons raw cacao powder, 1 scoop chocolate plant-based protein powder, 1 tablespoon almond butter, 1 cup unsweetened almond milk, 1 teaspoon cinnamon, 1 frozen banana, 1 tablespoon flaxseed meal
Servings: 2
Method of cooking: Blend
Procedure: 1. Place cacao and protein powder in blender; 2. Add almond butter; 3. Pour almond milk; 4. Sprinkle in cinnamon; 5. Add banana and flaxseed; 6. Blend until smooth and chocolaty.
Nutritional values: Estimated Calories: 330, Protein: 25g, Carbohydrates: 35g, Fat: 11g, Fiber: 10g.

Sunrise Citrus Smoothie

Preparation time: 5 minutes
Ingredients: 1 cup fresh orange juice, ½ cup carrot juice, ½ cup frozen mango, 1 tablespoon goji berries, 1 teaspoon turmeric root, grated, 1 tablespoon pumpkin seeds, 1 cup ice cubes
Servings: 2
Method of cooking: Blend
Procedure: 1. Blend orange juice and carrot juice together; 2. Add frozen mango and goji berries; 3. Grate in turmeric root; 4. Toss in pumpkin seeds; 5. Add ice cubes; 6. Blend until you achieve a sunrise-like blend.
Nutritional values: Estimated Calories: 180, Protein: 4g, Carbohydrates: 40g, Fat: 2g, Fiber: 3g.

Protein-Packed Breakfast Bowls

Quinoa and Berry Bowl

Preparation time: 20 minutes
Ingredients: 1 cup cooked quinoa, 1/2 cup strawberries, sliced, 1/2 cup blueberries, 1/4 cup raspberries, 2 tablespoons hemp seeds, 1 tablespoon honey, 1/2 cup almond milk
Servings: 2
Mode of cooking: Mix

Procedure: 1. Spoon quinoa into bowls; 2. Scatter berries over quinoa; 3. Sprinkle hemp seeds; 4. Drizzle with honey; 5. Pour almond milk around the edges.
Nutritional values: Approx. Calories: 320, Protein: 10g, Carbs: 55g, Fat: 8g, Fiber: 8g

Greek Yogurt and Granola Delight

Preparation time: 10 minutes
Ingredients: 1 cup Greek yogurt, 1/2 cup granola, 1 tablespoon chia seeds, 1/4 cup honey, 1/2 cup mixed nuts (almonds, walnuts, pistachios), chopped, 1/4 cup dried cherries
Servings: 2
Mode of cooking: Layer
Procedure: 1. Spread yogurt into bowls; 2. Sprinkle granola on top; 3. Distribute chia seeds; 4. Drizzle honey evenly; 5. Garnish with nuts and dried cherries.
Nutritional values: Approx. Calories: 450, Protein: 25g, Carbs: 36g, Fat: 22g, Fiber: 6g

Avocado and Egg Breakfast Bowl

Preparation time: 15 minutes
Ingredients: 2 eggs, poached, 1 avocado, sliced, 1/2 cup cooked black beans, 1/4 cup cherry tomatoes, halved, 2 tablespoons green onions, chopped, 1 tablespoon cilantro, chopped, 1 teaspoon lime juice, Salt and pepper to taste
Servings: 2
Mode of cooking: Assemble
Procedure: 1. Arrange avocado slices in bowls; 2. Place poached eggs next; 3. Spoon black beans around; 4. Dot with cherry tomatoes; 5. Sprinkle green onions and cilantro; 6. Squeeze lime juice over; 7. Season with salt and pepper.
Nutritional values: Approx. Calories: 350, Protein: 19g, Carbs: 22g, Fat: 23g, Fiber: 14g

Savory Breakfast Options

Spinach and Feta Omelette

Preparation time: 15 minutes
Ingredients: 3 large eggs, whisked, 1 cup fresh spinach, chopped, 1/4 cup feta cheese, crumbled, 1 tbsp olive oil, 1/4 tsp oregano, 1/4 tsp black pepper, 1/8 tsp sea salt

Servings: 1
Mode of cooking: Sauté and Fold
Procedure: 1. Heat olive oil in a pan; 2. Sauté spinach until wilted; 3. Pour eggs over spinach; 4. Sprinkle oregano, salt, and pepper; 5. Add feta before eggs set; 6. Fold omelette in half.
Nutritional values: Approx. Calories: 350, Protein: 22g, Carbs: 3g, Fat: 28g.

Turkey Sausage Breakfast Skillet

Preparation time: 25 minutes
Ingredients: 200g turkey sausage, sliced, 1/2 cup bell peppers, diced, 1/4 cup onions, diced, 1 garlic clove, minced, 2 medium potatoes, diced, 1 tbsp olive oil, 1/2 tsp paprika, Salt and pepper to taste
Servings: 2
Mode of cooking: Sauté
Procedure: 1. Brown sausage in skillet; 2. Remove sausage, sauté onions, garlic, bell peppers; 3. Add potatoes, cook until tender; 4. Stir in paprika; 5. Return sausage to skillet; 6. Season with salt and pepper.
Nutritional values: Approx. Calories: 400, Protein: 21g, Carbs: 38g, Fat: 20g.

Zucchini Hash Browns

Preparation time: 20 minutes
Ingredients: 2 cups zucchini, grated and drained, 1 egg, beaten, 1/4 cup whole wheat flour, 1/4 tsp garlic powder, 1/4 tsp onion powder, 2 tbsp olive oil, Salt and pepper to taste
Servings: 2

Mode of cooking: Fry
Procedure: 1. Combine zucchini, egg, flour, garlic and onion powder; 2. Heat oil in a pan; 3. Spoon mixture, press to flatten; 4. Fry until golden; 5. Flip once; 6. Season with salt and pepper.
Nutritional values: Approx. Calories: 230, Protein: 6g, Carbs: 18g, Fat: 16g.

Hearty Breakfast Bakes

Mushroom and Spinach Breakfast Casserole

Preparation time: 60 minutes
Ingredients: 1 lb sliced mushrooms, 2 cups fresh spinach, 6 beaten eggs, 1 cup grated cheddar cheese, 1/2 cup milk, 1 diced onion, 2 minced garlic cloves, 2 tbsp olive oil, 1 tsp thyme, Salt and pepper to taste
Servings: 4

Mode of cooking: Bake
Procedure: 1. Preheat oven to 375°F; 2. Sauté onions and garlic in oil; 3. Add mushrooms, cook until brown; 4. Stir in spinach until wilted; 5. Combine eggs, milk, cheese, thyme, salt, pepper; 6. Fold sautéed veggies into egg mixture; 7. Pour into greased baking dish; 8. Bake for 45 minutes.
Nutritional values: Approx. Calories: 300, Protein: 20g, Carbs: 6g, Fat: 22g.

Mini Breakfast Frittatas

Preparation time: 30 minutes
Ingredients: 8 eggs, 1/4 cup milk, 1/2 cup diced tomatoes, 1/2 cup chopped spinach, 1/4 cup grated Parmesan, 1/4 cup finely chopped basil, Salt and pepper to taste, Cooking spray
Servings: 12 mini frittatas
Mode of cooking: Bake
Procedure: 1. Preheat oven to 350°F; 2. Whisk eggs and milk; 3. Stir in tomatoes, spinach, Parmesan, basil, salt, pepper; 4. Spray muffin tin with cooking spray; 5. Pour mixture into muffin cups; 6. Bake for 20 minutes.
Nutritional values: Approx. per frittata: Calories: 90, Protein: 6g, Carbs: 2g, Fat: 6g.

Sweet Potato and Kale Breakfast Bake

Preparation time: 70 minutes
Ingredients: 2 large sweet potatoes, cubed, 2 cups kale, torn, 1/2 red onion, sliced, 6 eggs, 1/2 cup almond milk, 1 tsp smoked paprika, 1/2 tsp cumin, Olive oil for drizzling, Salt and pepper to taste
Servings: 6
Mode of cooking: Roast and Bake
Procedure: 1. Preheat oven to 400°F; 2. Toss sweet potatoes in oil, paprika, cumin, salt, pepper; 3. Roast for 30 minutes; 4. Reduce oven to 350°F; 5. Layer kale and onion on potatoes; 6. Whisk eggs and almond milk; 7. Pour over veggies; 8. Bake for 40 minutes.
Nutritional values: Approx. Calories: 220, Protein: 11g, Carbs: 20g, Fat: 11g.

Almond Butter and Banana Muffins

Preparation time: 35 minutes
Ingredients: 2 ripe bananas, mashed, 3/4 cup almond butter, 1/4 cup maple syrup, 2 eggs, 1/2 cup almond flour, 1/2 tsp baking soda, 1 tsp vanilla extract, A pinch of salt
Servings: 12 muffins
Mode of cooking: Bake
Procedure: 1. Preheat oven to 350°F; 2. Combine bananas, almond butter, maple syrup, eggs, vanilla; 3. Mix almond flour, baking soda, salt; 4. Blend dry into wet ingredients; 5. Spoon into muffin cups; 6. Bake for 20 minutes.
Nutritional values: Approx. per muffin: Calories: 180, Protein: 5g, Carbs: 14g, Fat: 12g.

Chapter 5: Nourishing Lunch Recipes

Vibrant Salad Bowls

Grilled Chicken Caesar Salad

Preparation time: 25 minutes
Ingredients: 2 boneless chicken breasts, 6 cups Romaine lettuce, 1 cup croutons, 1/2 cup shaved Parmesan, 1/2 cup Caesar dressing, 2 tbsp olive oil, 1 tbsp lemon juice, 1 minced garlic clove, Salt and black pepper to taste
Servings: 4
Mode of cooking: Grill
Procedure: 1. Marinate chicken in garlic, lemon juice, oil, salt, pepper for 15 minutes; 2. Grill chicken until cooked; 3. Chop Romaine, mix with croutons, Parmesan; 4. Slice chicken, place over salad; 5. Drizzle with dressing.
Nutritional values: Approx. Calories: 450, Protein: 35g, Carbs: 14g, Fat: 28g.

Tuna Nicoise Salad

Preparation time: 20 minutes
Ingredients: 4 cups mixed greens, 1 can of tuna in olive oil, drained, 4 boiled eggs, quartered, 1/2 cup cherry tomatoes, halved, 1/4 cup black olives, 12 steamed green beans, 2 tbsp extra virgin olive oil, 1 tbsp red wine vinegar, 1 tsp Dijon mustard, Salt and black pepper to taste
Servings: 4
Mode of cooking: Boil/Steam
Procedure: 1. Arrange greens on plates; 2. Top with flaked tuna, eggs, tomatoes, olives, beans; 3. Whisk olive oil, vinegar, mustard, salt, pepper; 4. Drizzle over salad.
Nutritional values: Approx. Calories: 310, Protein: 27g, Carbs: 8g, Fat: 18g.

Quinoa, Beet, and Goat Cheese Salad

Preparation time: 45 minutes
Ingredients: 1 cup quinoa, 2 medium beets, roasted and cubed, 1/2 cup crumbled goat cheese, 4 cups arugula, 1/4 cup chopped walnuts, 3 tbsp balsamic vinegar, 1 tbsp honey, 3 tbsp olive oil, Salt and black pepper to taste
Servings: 4
Mode of cooking: Roast/Boil
Procedure: 1. Cook quinoa as per package; 2. Toss arugula, beets, quinoa, cheese, nuts; 3. Combine vinegar, honey, oil, salt, pepper; 4. Dress salad before serving.
Nutritional values: Approx. Calories: 390, Protein: 14g, Carbs: 40g, Fat: 20g.

Southwest Chickpea Salad

Preparation time: 15 minutes
Ingredients: 2 cans chickpeas, drained, 1 cup corn kernels, 1 diced red bell pepper, 1 diced avocado, 1/2 cup chopped cilantro, 1 minced jalapeno, 2 limes, juiced, 2 tbsp olive oil, 1 tsp cumin, Salt and black pepper to taste
Servings: 4
Mode of cooking: Mix
Procedure: 1. In a bowl, combine chickpeas, corn, bell pepper, avocado, cilantro, jalapeno; 2. Whisk lime juice, oil, cumin, salt, pepper; 3. Toss salad with dressing.
Nutritional values: Approx. Calories: 340, Protein: 11g, Carbs: 45g, Fat: 14g.

Hearty Soups and Stews

Lentil and Vegetable Soup

Preparation time: 55 minutes
Ingredients: 1 cup brown lentils, 1 diced carrot, 1 diced celery stalk, 1 chopped onion, 2 minced garlic cloves, 1 diced tomato, 6 cups vegetable broth, 2 tbsp olive oil, 1 tsp smoked paprika, 1 bay leaf, Salt and pepper to taste

Servings: 6
Mode of cooking: Simmer
Procedure: 1. Sauté onion, carrot, celery, garlic in oil; 2. Add tomatoes, lentils, paprika, bay leaf, broth; 3. Boil then simmer for 45 minutes; 4. Season with salt, pepper.
Nutritional values: Approx. Calories: 240, Protein: 13g, Carbs: 35g, Fat: 5g.

Chicken and Wild Rice Soup

Preparation time: 1 hour and 10 minutes

Ingredients: 1 lb diced chicken breast, 1 cup wild rice, 1 diced onion, 2 diced carrots, 2 diced celery stalks, 6 cups chicken broth, 1 tsp thyme, 1 minced garlic clove, 2 tbsp unsalted butter, Salt and pepper to taste

Servings: 6

Mode of cooking: Sauté/Simmer

Procedure: 1. Sauté onion, garlic, carrots, celery in butter; 2. Add chicken, rice, thyme, broth; 3. Boil, reduce to simmer for 1 hour; 4. Season with salt, pepper.

Nutritional values: Approx. Calories: 300, Protein: 25g, Carbs: 40g, Fat: 6g.

Creamy Tomato and Basil Soup

Preparation time: 30 minutes

Ingredients: 2 cups crushed tomatoes, 1 cup heavy cream, 1 minced onion, 2 minced garlic cloves, 1/4 cup fresh basil, 1 tsp sugar, 2 tbsp olive oil, 3 cups vegetable broth, Salt and pepper to taste

Servings: 4

Mode of cooking: Blend/Simmer

Procedure: 1. Sauté onion, garlic in oil; 2. Add tomatoes, sugar, broth; 3. Simmer for 20 minutes; 4. Blend until smooth, return to heat; 5. Stir in cream, basil, season.

Nutritional values: Approx. Calories: 250, Protein: 3g, Carbs: 15g, Fat: 20g.

Spiced Pumpkin Soup

Preparation time: 45 minutes

Ingredients: 2 cups pumpkin puree, 1 diced onion, 1 minced garlic clove, 4 cups vegetable broth, 1 cup light cream, 1 tsp cinnamon, 1/4 tsp nutmeg, 2 tbsp maple syrup, 1 tbsp olive oil, Salt and pepper to taste

Servings: 4

Mode of cooking: Sauté/Simmer

Procedure: 1. Sauté onion, garlic in oil; 2. Stir in pumpkin, cinnamon, nutmeg, syrup, broth; 3. Simmer for 30 minutes; 4. Blend until smooth; 5. Mix in cream, heat through, season.

Nutritional values: Approx. Calories: 220, Protein: 4g, Carbs: 25g, Fat: 12g.

Protein-Packed Wraps and Sandwiches

Turkey and Avocado Wrap

Preparation time: 15 minutes
Ingredients: 2 whole wheat tortillas, 1 ripe avocado (sliced), 6 oz sliced smoked turkey breast, 1/4 cup alfalfa sprouts, 1 diced tomato, 2 tbsp tzatziki sauce, 1/2 cup chopped romaine lettuce, Salt and pepper to taste
Servings: 2
Mode of cooking: Assembly
Procedure: 1. Lay tortillas flat; 2. Spread tzatziki; 3. Layer turkey, avocado, tomato, lettuce, sprouts; 4. Season; 5. Roll tightly, slice in half.
Nutritional values: Approx. Calories: 350, Protein: 25g, Carbs: 35g, Fat: 15g.

Grilled Vegetable and Hummus Wrap

Preparation time: 20 minutes
Ingredients: 2 spinach tortillas, 1/2 zucchini (sliced & grilled), 1/2 red bell pepper (sliced & grilled), 1/4 red onion (sliced & grilled), 4 tbsp hummus, 1/2 cup mixed greens, 1 tbsp balsamic glaze, Salt and pepper to taste
Servings: 2
Mode of cooking: Grill/Assembly
Procedure: 1. Grill veggies; 2. Spread hummus on tortillas; 3. Arrange veggies, greens; 4. Drizzle glaze, season; 5. Roll, slice.
Nutritional values: Approx. Calories: 320, Protein: 8g, Carbs: 45g, Fat: 13g.

Tofu Lettuce Wraps

Preparation time: 25 minutes
Ingredients: 1 lb firm tofu (crumbled), 1 head butter lettuce, 2 tbsp soy sauce, 1 tbsp sesame oil, 1 tsp chili flakes, 1 minced garlic clove, 1/2 cup diced water chestnuts, 1/4 cup green onions (sliced), 1 tsp ginger (grated), Salt to taste
Servings: 4
Mode of cooking: Sauté/Assembly
Procedure: 1. Sauté tofu, garlic, ginger; 2. Add soy sauce, sesame oil, chili; 3. Mix in chestnuts, onions; 4. Spoon into lettuce leaves.
Nutritional values: Approx. Calories: 150, Protein: 10g, Carbs: 8g, Fat: 9g.

Roast Beef and Horseradish Sandwich

Preparation time: 10 minutes
Ingredients: 4 slices rye bread, 8 oz thin-sliced roast beef, 2 tbsp horseradish sauce, 1/4 cup arugula, 1 tbsp stone-ground mustard, 2 slices Swiss cheese, 1/4 red onion (thinly sliced), Salt and pepper to taste
Servings: 2

Mode of cooking: Assembly
Procedure: 1. Spread mustard, horseradish on bread; 2. Layer beef, onion, cheese, arugula; 3. Season; 4. Close sandwiches, cut diagonally.
Nutritional values: Approx. Calories: 380, Protein: 30g, Carbs: 30g, Fat: 15g.

Main Course Delights

Seared Salmon with Asparagus

Preparation time: 22 minutes
Ingredients: 2 salmon fillets (6 oz each), 1 bunch asparagus, 1 tbsp olive oil, 1 tsp grated lemon zest, 1 tbsp lemon juice, Salt and freshly ground black pepper, 1 tsp dill
Servings: 2
Mode of cooking: Pan-sear/Sauté
Procedure: 1. Season salmon; 2. Heat oil, sear salmon skin-side down until crisp; 3. Flip, cook to desired doneness; 4. Blanch asparagus; 5. Sauté asparagus in remaining oil, season with lemon, dill.
Nutritional values: Approx. Calories: 300, Protein: 34g, Carbs: 6g, Fat: 16g.

Turkey Meatball Zoodles

Preparation time: 35 minutes
Ingredients: 1 lb ground turkey, 1/4 cup breadcrumbs, 1 egg, 2 minced garlic cloves, 1/4 cup chopped parsley, Salt and pepper, 3 zucchinis (spiraled), 1 tbsp olive oil, 1 cup marinara sauce
Servings: 4
Mode of cooking: Bake/Sauté
Procedure: 1. Mix turkey, breadcrumbs, egg, garlic, parsley, season; 2. Form meatballs, bake at 375°F for 20 minutes; 3. Sauté zoodles in oil; 4. Heat sauce, combine with meatballs, serve over zoodles.
Nutritional values: Approx. Calories: 280, Protein: 27g, Carbs: 14g, Fat: 14g.

Veggie-Stuffed Bell Peppers

Preparation time: 45 minutes
Ingredients: 4 bell peppers (halved), 1 cup cooked quinoa, 1 diced onion, 1/2 cup corn, 1/2 cup black beans, 1/2 cup diced tomatoes, 1 tsp cumin, Salt and pepper, 1/2 cup shredded cheddar cheese
Servings: 4
Mode of cooking: Bake
Procedure: 1. Preheat oven to 350°F; 2. Mix quinoa, onion, corn, beans, tomatoes, cumin, season; 3. Stuff peppers, top with cheese; 4. Bake 25 minutes.
Nutritional values: Approx. Calories: 220, Protein: 10g, Carbs: 30g, Fat: 7g.

Spinach and Feta Stuffed Chicken Breast

Preparation time: 30 minutes
Ingredients: 2 large chicken breasts, 1 cup chopped spinach, 1/2 cup crumbled feta, 1 minced garlic clove, Salt and pepper, 1 tbsp olive oil, 1 tsp paprika
Servings: 2
Mode of cooking: Sauté/Bake
Procedure: 1. Preheat to 375°F; 2. Cut a pocket in chicken; 3. Mix spinach, feta, garlic, stuff chicken; 4. Season outside, sear in pan, bake 20 min.
Nutritional values: Approx. Calories: 360, Protein: 55g, Carbs: 4g, Fat: 14g.

Portobello Mushroom Caps with Quinoa Filling

Preparation time: 40 minutes
Ingredients: 4 large portobello mushroom caps, 1 cup cooked quinoa, 1/4 cup pine nuts, 1/4 cup sundried tomatoes (chopped), 1/4 cup crumbled goat cheese, 1 tbsp chopped basil, Salt and pepper, 1 tbsp balsamic reduction
Servings: 4
Mode of cooking: Bake
Procedure: 1. Preheat to 375°F; 2. Remove mushroom stems, season caps; 3. Combine quinoa, nuts, tomatoes, basil, goat cheese; 4. Stuff mushrooms, drizzle with balsamic, bake 20 min.
Nutritional values: Approx. Calories: 250, Protein: 10g, Carbs: 20g, Fat: 15g.

Chapter 6: Delicious Dinner Delicacies

Flavorful Stir-Fries

Shrimp and Broccoli Stir-Fry

Preparation time: 25 minutes
Ingredients: Ingr. 1 lb shrimp (peeled and deveined), 2 cups broccoli florets, 1 tbsp vegetable oil, 2 tsp Szechuan sauce, 1 tsp minced garlic, 1 tsp cornstarch dissolved in 2 tbsp water
Servings: 4
Method of cooking: Wok-fry
Procedure: 1. Blanch broccoli; 2. Heat oil, garlic, add shrimp; 3. Stir-fry shrimp until pink; 4. Add broccoli, Szechuan sauce; 5. Thicken with cornstarch mixture.
Nutritional values: Approx. Calories: 180, Protein: 23g, Carbs: 8g, Fat: 6g.

Chicken Teriyaki with Mixed Vegetables

Preparation time: 30 minutes
Ingredients: Ingr. 2 chicken breasts (sliced), 2 tbsp teriyaki glaze, 1 tbsp sesame seeds, 1 cup mixed bell peppers, sliced, 1/2 cup sliced zucchini, 1/2 cup sliced onions, 1 tbsp canola oil
Servings: 4
Method of cooking: Wok-fry
Procedure: 1. Marinate chicken in teriyaki; 2. Sear chicken in oil; 3. Add vegetables; 4. Cook until veggies are tender; 5. Sprinkle sesame seeds.
Nutritional values: Approx. Calories: 220, Protein: 26g, Carbs: 12g, Fat: 7g.

Beef and Snow Pea Stir-Fry

Preparation time: 25 minutes
Ingredients: Ingr. 1 lb beef strips, 2 tbsp hoisin sauce, 1 tsp grated ginger, 1 cup snow peas, 1/2 cup sliced red onions, 2 tbsp peanut oil, 1 tsp sesame oil, 1 tbsp soy sauce
Servings: 4
Method of cooking: Wok-fry
Procedure: 1. Toss beef with soy and ginger; 2. Heat peanut oil, brown beef; 3. Add snow peas, onions; 4. Drizzle with hoisin, sesame oil.
Nutritional values: Approx. Calories: 290, Protein: 25g, Carbs: 10g, Fat: 16g.

Tofu and Bell Pepper Stir-Fry

Preparation time: 25 minutes
Ingredients: Ingr. 14 oz firm tofu (cubed and dried), 2 cups mixed bell peppers (chopped), 1 tbsp coconut oil, 2 tsp tamari, 1 tsp chili flakes, 1 tbsp maple syrup, 1 tsp apple cider vinegar
Servings: 4

Method of cooking: Wok-fry
Procedure: 1. Fry tofu until golden; 2. Remove, sauté peppers in coconut oil; 3. Return tofu, season with tamari, chili, syrup, vinegar.
Nutritional values: Approx. Calories: 150, Protein: 10g, Carbs: 11g, Fat: 8g

Grilled Perfections

Grilled Lemon Herb Chicken

- **Preparation time**: 1 hour (includes marinating time)
- **Ingredients**: 4 boneless chicken breasts, 2 tbsp olive oil, zest of 1 lemon, 2 tbsp lemon juice, 3 tbsp chopped fresh thyme, 1 tbsp minced garlic, salt to taste, ground black pepper to taste
- **Servings**: 4
- **Method of cooking**: Grill
- **Procedure**: 1. Flatten chicken to even thickness; 2. Whisk together oil, lemon zest, juice, thyme, garlic, salt, pepper; 3. Marinate chicken for 30 mins; 4. Preheat grill to medium-high; 5. Grill chicken 6-7 mins each side.
- **Nutritional values**: Approx. Calories: 210, Protein: 35g, Carbs: 1g, Fat: 7g.

Seared Tuna Steaks

- **Preparation time**: 25 minutes
- **Ingredients**: 4 tuna steaks (1-inch thick), 2 tbsp soy sauce, 1 tbsp lime juice, 1 tbsp olive oil, 1 tsp honey, 1 tsp red chili flakes, 1 tsp grated ginger, lime slices for garnish
- **Servings**: 4
- **Method of cooking**: Sear
- **Procedure**: 1. Whisk soy sauce, lime juice, oil, honey, chili, ginger; 2. Coat tuna steaks, let sit 10 mins; 3. Preheat grill to high; 4. Sear tuna 1-2 mins each side; 5. Serve with lime slices.
- **Nutritional values**: Approx. Calories: 180, Protein: 40g, Carbs: 2g, Fat: 2g.

Herb-Crusted Lamb Chops

- **Preparation time**: 35 minutes (includes resting time)
- **Ingredients**: 8 lamb chops, 1/4 cup bread crumbs, 2 tbsp chopped rosemary, 4 cloves garlic minced, 2 tbsp Dijon mustard, salt and black pepper to taste, 2 tbsp olive oil
- **Servings**: 4
- **Method of cooking**: Grill
- **Procedure**: 1. Mix bread crumbs, rosemary, garlic, salt, pepper; 2. Brush chops with mustard; 3. Press crumb mixture onto chops; 4. Preheat grill to medium; 5. Grill 4-5 mins per side; 6. Rest meat 5 mins before serving.
- **Nutritional values**: Approx. Calories: 310, Protein: 24g, Carbs: 5g, Fat: 22g.

- **Ingredients**: 2 medium eggplants sliced, 2 large zucchinis sliced, 1/4 cup balsamic vinegar, 3 tbsp olive oil, 2 cloves garlic minced, 1 tsp mixed Italian herbs, salt and pepper to taste
- **Servings**: 4
- **Method of cooking**: Grill
- **Procedure**: 1. Whisk balsamic, oil, garlic, herbs, salt, pepper; 2. Brush slices with mixture; 3. Preheat grill to medium-high; 4. Grill vegetables 3-4 mins each side.
- **Nutritional values**: Approx. Calories: 120, Protein: 3g, Carbs: 15g, Fat: 7g.

Grilled Eggplant and Zucchini Slices

- **Preparation time**: 20 minutes

Oven-Baked Wonders

Rosemary Garlic Roast Beef

- **Preparation time**: 1 hour and 30 minutes
- **Ingredients**: 1 (3-pound) beef round roast, 4 tbsp fresh rosemary minced, 6 cloves garlic minced, 2 tbsp olive oil, 1 tbsp coarse sea salt, 1 tsp cracked black pepper, 2 tbsp balsamic vinegar
- **Servings**: 6
- **Method of cooking**: Roasting
- **Procedure**: 1. Preheat oven to 375°F (190°C); 2. Mix rosemary, garlic, oil, vinegar, salt, pepper; 3. Rub mixture on beef; 4. Place in roasting pan; 5. Roast until desired doneness; 6. Rest before slicing.
- **Nutritional values**: Approx. Calories: 450, Protein: 60g, Carbs: 1g, Fat: 22g.

Baked Tilapia with Dill Sauce

- **Preparation time**: 25 minutes

- **Ingredients**: 4 tilapia fillets, 2 tbsp melted unsalted butter, 1 lemon zest and juice, 2 tbsp fresh dill chopped, 1 clove garlic minced, salt to taste, ground white pepper to taste, lemon slices for serving
- **Servings**: 4
- **Method of cooking**: Baking
- **Procedure**: 1. Preheat oven to 400°F (200°C); 2. Whisk butter, lemon zest, juice, dill, garlic, salt, pepper; 3. Place fillets in baking dish; 4. Pour mixture over tilapia; 5. Bake 12-15 minutes; 6. Serve with lemon slices.

Herb and Parmesan Crusted Cod

- **Preparation time**: 30 minutes

- **Ingredients**: 4 cod fillets, 1/2 cup grated Parmesan cheese, 1/4 cup finely chopped parsley, 1 tbsp chopped oregano, 1 tsp garlic powder, 2 tbsp olive oil, salt and pepper to taste, lemon wedges for serving
- **Servings**: 4
- **Method of cooking**: Baking
- **Procedure**: 1. Preheat oven to 400°F (200°C); 2. Combine Parmesan, parsley, oregano, garlic powder, salt, pepper; 3. Brush fillets with oil; 4. Coat with cheese mixture; 5. Place on baking sheet; 6. Bake 15-20 minutes; 7. Serve with lemon.
- **Nutritional values**: Approx. Calories: 180, Protein: 34g, Carbs: 1g, Fat: 5g.

- **Nutritional values**: Approx. Calories: 220, Protein: 38g, Carbs: 2g, Fat: 7g.

One-Pot Meals

Vegetarian Chili

- **Preparation time**: 40 minutes

- **Ingredients**: 1 tbsp olive oil, 1 large onion chopped, 2 bell peppers diced, 3 cloves garlic minced, 2 carrots diced, 2 celery stalks diced, 1 zucchini diced, 1 cup sweet corn, 2 tbsp tomato paste, 1 can diced tomatoes, 1 can black beans drained, 1 can kidney beans drained, 1 can cannellini beans drained, 1 tsp smoked paprika, 1 tsp cumin, 1 tsp chili powder, salt and pepper to taste, 2 cups vegetable broth, fresh cilantro for garnish
- **Servings**: 6

- **Method of cooking**: Simmering
- **Procedure**: 1. Heat oil in a pot; 2. Sauté onion, garlic, peppers, carrots, celery; 3. Add zucchini, corn, cook 5 min; 4. Stir in tomato paste, diced tomatoes, beans, spices; 5. Pour in broth; 6. Simmer 25 min; 7. Garnish with cilantro.
- **Nutritional values**: Approx. Calories: 210, Protein: 10g, Carbs: 40g, Fat: 3g.

Beef and Vegetable Stew

- **Preparation time**: 2 hours
- **Ingredients**: 1.5 lbs beef chuck cut into cubes, 1 tbsp vegetable oil, 3 carrots sliced, 2 potatoes diced, 1 onion chopped, 2 celery stalks sliced, 3 cloves garlic minced, 1 tsp thyme, 1 tsp rosemary, 1 bay leaf, 2 tbsp flour, 4 cups beef broth, salt and pepper to taste
- **Servings**: 6
- **Method of cooking**: Braising
- **Procedure**: 1. Brown beef in oil; 2. Add onion, garlic, sauté; 3. Sprinkle flour, cook 2 min; 4. Add broth, carrots, potatoes, celery, herbs; 5. Bring to boil, then simmer 1.5 hrs; 6. Season to taste.
- **Nutritional values**: Approx. Calories: 330, Protein: 26g, Carbs: 24g, Fat: 15g.

Spaghetti Squash Primavera

- **Preparation time**: 1 hour
- **Ingredients**: 1 spaghetti squash halved, seeds removed, 1 tbsp olive oil, 1 zucchini sliced, 1 bell pepper diced, 1 carrot julienned, 1/2 cup cherry tomatoes halved, 2 cloves garlic minced, 1 tsp Italian seasoning, salt and pepper to taste, fresh basil for garnish, grated Parmesan cheese for serving
- **Servings**: 4
- **Method of cooking**: Roasting and Sautéing
- **Procedure**: 1. Roast squash 40 min at 375°F; 2. Sauté garlic, zucchini, pepper, carrot; 3. Add tomatoes, seasoning; 4. Fork squash strands into vegetables; 5. Top with basil, Parmesan.
- **Nutritional values**: Approx. Calories: 150, Protein: 4g, Carbs: 27g, Fat: 5g.

Chicken and Vegetable Curry

- **Preparation time**: 30 minutes
- **Ingredients**: 1 lb chicken breast cut into pieces, 1 tbsp coconut oil, 1 onion diced, 2 cloves garlic minced, 1 bell pepper diced, 1 cup broccoli florets, 1 tbsp curry powder, 1 tsp turmeric, 1 can coconut milk, 1/2 cup chicken broth, salt to taste, cilantro for garnish

- **Servings**: 4
- **Method of cooking**: Simmering
- **Procedure**: 1. Heat oil, cook chicken; 2. Add onion, garlic, bell pepper, broccoli; 3. Stir in curry, turmeric; 4. Pour coconut milk, broth; 5. Simmer 20 min; 6. Garnish with cilantro.

- **Nutritional values**: Approx. Calories: 290, Protein: 28g, Carbs: 8g, Fat: 17g.

Global Delights

Thai Green Chicken Curry

- **Preparation time**: 30 minutes
- **Ingredients**: 1 tbsp coconut oil, 1 lb chicken breast sliced, 2 tbsp green curry paste, 1 can (14 oz) coconut milk, 1/2 cup chicken broth, 1 cup bamboo shoots, 1 bell pepper sliced, 1 zucchini sliced, 1 tbsp fish sauce, 1 tsp palm sugar, basil leaves for garnish, steamed jasmine rice for serving
- **Servings**: 4
- **Mode of cooking**: Simmering
- **Procedure**: 1. Heat oil, cook chicken until white; 2. Add curry paste, sauté; 3. Pour coconut milk, broth, simmer; 4. Add bamboo, bell pepper, zucchini, cook until tender; 5. Season with fish sauce, palm sugar; 6. Garnish with basil, serve with rice.
- **Nutritional values**: Approx. Calories: 360, Protein: 25g, Carbs: 15g, Fat: 22g.

Mediterranean Chickpea Stew

- **Preparation time**: 25 minutes
- **Ingredients**: 2 tbsp olive oil, 1 onion diced, 2 cloves garlic minced, 1 tsp cumin, 1 tsp paprika, 1 can (14 oz) diced tomatoes, 2 cans (14 oz each) chickpeas drained, 4 cups fresh spinach, 1/2 cup vegetable broth, salt and pepper to taste, lemon wedges for serving
- **Servings**: 4
- **Method of cooking**: Stewing
- **Procedure**: 1. Heat oil, cook onion, garlic; 2. Stir in spices; 3. Add tomatoes, chickpeas, cook 10 min; 4. Put spinach, pour broth, simmer until wilted; 5. Season, serve with lemon.
- **Nutritional values**: Approx. Calories: 250, Protein: 9g, Carbs: 35g, Fat: 8g.

Italian Eggplant Parmesan

- **Preparation time**: 1 hour
- **Ingredients**: 2 eggplants sliced, 2 cups marinara sauce, 2 cups shredded mozzarella, 1/2 cup grated Parmesan, 1/4 cup basil leaves, 1/2 cup flour, 2 eggs beaten, 1 cup breadcrumbs, olive oil for frying, salt and pepper to taste
- **Servings**: 6
- **Method of cooking**: Baking and Frying
- **Procedure**: 1. Salt eggplant, rest 20 min, rinse; 2. Dredge in flour, egg, breadcrumbs; 3. Fry until golden, drain; 4. Layer eggplant, sauce, cheeses in baking dish; 5. Bake at 375°F for 25 min; 6. Top with basil.
- **Nutritional values**: Approx. Calories: 320, Protein: 18g, Carbs: 28g, Fat: 16g.

Mexican Stuffed Peppers

- **Preparation time**: 45 minutes
- **Ingredients**: 4 bell peppers halved, 1 lb ground beef, 1 cup cooked rice, 1 can (14 oz) black beans drained, 1 cup corn, 1 cup salsa, 1 tsp chili powder, 1 tsp cumin, 2 cups shredded cheddar cheese, fresh cilantro for garnish
- **Servings**: 8
- **Method of cooking**: Baking
- **Procedure**: 1. Preheat oven to 350°F; 2. Cook beef, season; 3. Combine rice, beans, corn, salsa, spices; 4. Stuff peppers, top with cheese; 5. Bake 30 min; 6. Garnish with cilantro.
- **Nutritional values**: Approx. Calories: 350, Protein: 22g, Carbs: 28g, Fat: 18g.

Chapter 7: Snack Time and Side Dishes

Healthy Snack Options

Almond & Chia Seed Energy Balls

- **Preparation time**: 15 minutes + 30 minutes chilling
- **Ingredients**: 1 cup raw almonds, 1/4 cup chia seeds, 1/2 cup shredded coconut, 1/4 cup honey, 1/2 cup peanut butter, 1 tsp vanilla extract
- **Servings**: 12 balls
- **Mode of cooking**: No cook, chill
- **Procedure**: 1. Pulse almonds to a coarse meal; 2. Mix with chia, coconut; 3. Stir in honey, peanut butter, vanilla; 4. Roll into balls; 5. Chill.
- **Nutritional values**: Approx. per ball: Calories: 120, Protein: 4g, Carbs: 8g, Fat: 9g.

Greek Yogurt Parfait with Fresh Berries

- **Preparation time**: 10 minutes
- **Ingredients**: 2 cups Greek yogurt, 1/2 cup granola, 1 cup mixed berries, 2 tbsp honey, 1/4 tsp cinnamon
- **Servings**: 2
- **Method of cooking**: Layered assembly
- **Procedure**: 1. Spoon yogurt into glasses; 2. Add granola layer; 3. Top with berries; 4. Drizzle honey; 5. Sprinkle cinnamon.
- **Nutritional values**: Approx. per serving: Calories: 220, Protein: 15g, Carbs: 25g, Fat: 6g.

Spinach and Artichoke Dip

- **Preparation time**: 20 minutes + 25 minutes baking
- **Ingredients**: 1 cup cooked spinach, 1 cup chopped artichokes, 1/2 cup sour cream, 1/4 cup mayonnaise, 1/2 cup grated Parmesan, 1/2 cup shredded mozzarella, 1 clove garlic minced, salt and pepper to taste
- **Servings**: 4

- **Method of cooking**: Baking
- **Procedure**: 1. Combine spinach, artichokes, creams, cheeses, garlic; 2. Season; 3. Transfer to baking dish; 4. Bake at 375°F until bubbly.
- **Nutritional values**: Approx. per serving: Calories: 220, Protein: 8g, Carbs: 10g, Fat: 16g.

Baked Zucchini Fries with Avocado Dip

- **Preparation time**: 15 minutes + 20 minutes baking
- **Ingredients**: 2 zucchinis cut into fries, 1 cup panko breadcrumbs, 1/4 cup grated Parmesan, 1 egg, salt and pepper to taste; **Dip**: 1 ripe avocado, 1/2 cup Greek yogurt, 1 tbsp lime juice, 1 clove garlic minced
- **Servings**: 4
- **Method of cooking**: Baking
- **Procedure**: 1. Coat zucchini in egg, panko, Parmesan; 2. Season; 3. Bake at 425°F until crispy; **Dip**: Blend avocado, yogurt, lime, garlic.
- **Nutritional values**: Approx. per serving (including dip): Calories: 180, Protein: 8g, Carbs: 20g, Fat: 8g.

Roasted Chickpeas with Turmeric and Cumin

- **Preparation time**: 10 minutes + 40 minutes roasting
- **Ingredients**: 2 cups canned chickpeas drained, 1 tbsp olive oil, 1 tsp turmeric, 1 tsp cumin, salt to taste
- **Servings**: 4
- **Method of cooking**: Roasting
- **Procedure**: 1. Toss chickpeas with oil, spices; 2. Spread on baking sheet; 3. Roast at 400°F turning occasionally until crunchy.
- **Nutritional values**: Approx. per serving: Calories: 150, Protein: 6g, Carbs: 20g, Fat: 6g.

Celery Sticks with Almond Butter Drizzle

- **Preparation time**: 10 minutes
- **Ingredients**: 5 celery stalks, 1/2 cup smooth almond butter, 1 tbsp honey, 1/4 tsp ground cinnamon, 1 tbsp sliced almonds for garnish
- **Servings**: 5
- **Mode of cooking**: No cook, drizzle
- **Procedure**: 1. Wash and cut celery into 3-inch sticks; 2. Mix almond butter with honey and cinnamon; 3. Drizzle almond butter mix over celery; 4. Garnish with sliced almonds.

- **Nutritional values**: Approx. per serving: Calories: 150, Protein: 4g, Carbs: 8g, Fat: 12g.

Fresh Spring Rolls with Peanut Sauce

- **Preparation time**: 30 minutes
- **Ingredients**: 10 rice paper wrappers, 1 cup mixed lettuce, 1/2 cup mint leaves, 1/2 cup cilantro, 1 carrot julienned, 1 cucumber julienned, 1/2 red bell pepper julienned; **Sauce**: 1/4 cup peanut butter, 2 tbsp soy sauce, 1 tbsp lime juice, 1 tsp honey, 1 tsp grated ginger, water to thin
- **Servings**: 10 rolls
- **Method of cooking**: Assemble, blend for sauce
- **Procedure**: 1. Soften rice papers; 2. Lay on lettuce, herbs, veggies; 3. Roll tightly; **Sauce**: Blend peanut butter, soy, lime, honey, ginger.
- **Nutritional values**: Approx. per roll (with sauce): Calories: 100, Protein: 3g, Carbs: 15g, Fat: 3.5g.

Baked Kale Chips

- **Preparation time**: 10 minutes + 15 minutes baking
- **Ingredients**: 1 bunch kale, 1 tbsp olive oil, 1/2 tsp garlic powder, salt to taste
- **Servings**: 4
- **Method of cooking**: Baking

- **Procedure**: 1. Tear kale into bite-size pieces; 2. Toss with oil, garlic powder, salt; 3. Bake at 350°F until edges brown but not burnt.
- **Nutritional values**: Approx. per serving: Calories: 58, Protein: 2g, Carbs: 7g, Fat: 3g.

Edamame Beans with Sea Salt

- **Preparation time**: 5 minutes + 5 minutes cooking
- **Ingredients**: 2 cups frozen edamame in pods, 1 tsp sea salt flakes
- **Servings**: 4
- **Method of cooking**: Boil
- **Procedure**: 1. Boil edamame until tender; 2. Drain and sprinkle with sea salt.
- **Nutritional values**: Approx. per serving: Calories: 100, Protein: 9g, Carbs: 8g, Fat: 3g.

Cottage Cheese Cups with Pineapple Chunks

- **Preparation time**: 5 minutes
- **Ingredients**: 2 cups cottage cheese, 1 cup pineapple chunks, 1 tbsp shredded coconut, 1 tsp chia seeds
- **Servings**: 4
- **Method of cooking**: No cook, assemble
- **Procedure**: 1. Divide cottage cheese into cups; 2. Top with pineapple; 3. Sprinkle coconut and chia seeds.
- **Nutritional values**: Approx. per serving: Calories: 150, Protein: 14g, Carbs: 10g, Fat: 5g.

Vegetable Sides to Love

Maple Glazed Brussels Sprouts

- **Preparation time**: 25 minutes
- **Ingredients**: 1 lb Brussels sprouts (halved), 3 tbsp maple syrup, 2 tbsp olive oil, 1/4 tsp crushed red pepper, salt to taste
- **Servings**: 4
- **Method of cooking**: Roasting
- **Procedure**: 1. Preheat oven to 400°F; 2. Toss Brussels sprouts with maple syrup, olive oil, red pepper, and salt; 3. Spread on baking sheet; 4. Roast until caramelized, about 20 minutes.
- **Nutritional values:** Approx. per serving: Calories: 140, Protein: 3g, Carbs: 17g, Fat. 7g.

Cauliflower and Cheese Gratin

- **Preparation time**: 35 minutes
- **Ingredients**: 1 large cauliflower (cut into florets), 2 cups shredded cheddar cheese, 1/4 cup cream, 1 garlic clove minced, 1/2 tsp nutmeg, salt, and pepper to taste
- **Servings**: 6
- **Method of cooking**: Baking

- **Procedure**: 1. Preheat oven to 375°F; 2. Steam cauliflower until tender; 3. In a bowl, mix cheese, cream, garlic, nutmeg; 4. Layer cauliflower in baking dish, pour cheese mixture; 5. Bake until golden, 15 minutes.
- **Nutritional values**: Calories: 200, Protein: 12g, Carbs: 10g, Fat: 14g

Sweet Potato Wedges with Cilantro Dip

- **Preparation time**: 30 minutes
- **Ingredients**: 2 large sweet potatoes (cut into wedges), 2 tbsp olive oil, salt, pepper; **Dip**: 1 cup Greek yogurt, 1/4 cup chopped cilantro, 1 tbsp lime juice, 1 tsp honey
- **Servings**: 4
- **Method of cooking**: Baking
- **Procedure**: 1. Preheat oven to 425°F; 2. Toss wedges with oil, salt, pepper; 3. Bake until crispy, 25 minutes; **Dip**: Mix yogurt, cilantro, lime, honey.
- **Nutritional values**: Calories: 230, Protein: 5g, Carbs: 35g, Fat: 7g

Lemon Butter Broccoli Florets

- **Preparation time**: 15 minutes

- **Ingredients**: 1 lb broccoli florets, 2 tbsp butter, 1 tbsp lemon juice, 1 tsp lemon zest, salt, and black pepper to taste
- **Servings**: 4
- **Method of cooking**: Sautéing
- **Procedure**: 1. Steam broccoli until tender; 2. In a pan, melt butter, add lemon juice, zest; 3. Toss broccoli in lemon butter, season.
- **Nutritional values**: Calories: 80, Protein: 3g, Carbs: 6g, Fat: 5g

Grilled Corn with Herb Butter

- **Preparation time**: 20 minutes
- **Ingredients**: 4 ears of corn, husked; **Herb Butter**: 4 tbsp butter (softened), 1 tbsp chopped parsley, 1 tbsp chopped chives, 1 tsp garlic powder, salt
- **Servings**: 4
- **Method of cooking**: Grilling
- **Procedure**: 1. Grill corn until charred, 10 minutes; 2. Mix butter with parsley, chives, garlic, salt; 3. Brush herb butter on grilled corn.
- **Nutritional values**: Calories: 150, Protein: 3g, Carbs: 17g, Fat: 9g

Grilled Corn with Herb Butter

- **Preparation time**: 20 minutes
- **Ingredients**: 4 ears corn, husked; Herb Butter: 4 tbsp softened butter, 1 tbsp chopped parsley, 1 tsp minced garlic, salt
- **Servings**: 4
- **Method of cooking**: Grilling
- **Procedure**: 1. Grill corn until tender and charred, 10-15 mins; 2. Mix butter, parsley, garlic, and salt; 3. Brush herb butter on corn.
- **Nutritional values**: Calories: 160, Fat: 9g, Carbs: 18g, Protein: 3g

Green Beans Almondine

- **Preparation time**: 15 minutes
- **Ingredients**: 1 lb green beans, trimmed, 2 tbsp sliced almonds, 2 tbsp butter, 1 tsp lemon juice, salt, pepper
- **Servings**: 4
- **Method of cooking**: Sautéing
- **Procedure**: 1. Blanch green beans; 2. Sauté almonds in butter until golden; 3. Add green beans, lemon juice; season.
- **Nutritional values**: Calories: 100, Fat: 7g, Carbs: 8g, Protein: 3g

Roasted Beets with Feta Crumble

- **Preparation time**: 45 minutes

- **Ingredients**: 4 medium beets, 1/4 cup crumbled feta cheese, 2 tbsp olive oil, 1 tbsp balsamic vinegar, salt, pepper
- **Servings**: 4
- **Method of cooking**: Roasting
- **Procedure**: 1. Roast beets until tender, 40 mins; 2. Slice beets, top with feta; 3. Drizzle oil, vinegar; season.
- **Nutritional values**: Calories: 120, Fat: 7g, Carbs: 10g, Protein: 4g

Spinach and Garlic Sauté

- **Preparation time**: 10 minutes
- **Ingredients**: 1 lb spinach, 3 garlic cloves minced, 2 tbsp olive oil, salt, pepper, lemon zest
- **Servings**: 4
- **Method of cooking**: Sautéing
- **Procedure**: 1. Heat oil, sauté garlic until fragrant; 2. Add spinach, cook until wilted; 3. Season, add lemon zest.
- **Nutritional values**: Calories: 60, Fat: 5g, Carbs: 3g, Protein: 2g

Mediterranean Stuffed Tomatoes

- **Preparation time**: 30 minutes
- **Ingredients**: 4 large tomatoes, hollowed; Filling: 1 cup cooked quinoa, 1/2 cup chopped olives, 1/4 cup crumbled feta, 2 tbsp chopped parsley, 1 tbsp olive oil, salt, pepper
- **Servings**: 4
- **Method of cooking**: Baking
- **Procedure**: 1. Preheat oven to 375°F; 2. Mix filling ingredients; 3. Stuff tomatoes, bake 20 mins.
- **Nutritional values**: Calories: 150, Fat: 8g, Carbs: 16g, Protein:
- 5g

Wholesome Grains and Legumes

Quinoa Tabbouleh Salad

- **Preparation time**: 20 minutes
- **Ingredients**: 1 cup quinoa cooked, 1 large cucumber diced, 2 tomatoes diced, 1/2 cup parsley chopped, 1/4 cup lemon juice, 3 tbsp olive oil, salt, pepper
- **Servings**: 4
- **Mode of cooking**: Mixing
- **Procedure**: 1. Combine quinoa, cucumber, tomatoes, parsley; 2. Add lemon juice, olive oil, salt, pepper; mix well.

-

- **Nutritional values**: Calories: 210, Fat: 10g, Carbs: 27g, Protein: 6g

Lentil and Tomato Stew

- **Preparation time**: 45 minutes
- **Ingredients**: 1 cup lentils, 1 can diced tomatoes, 1 onion diced, 2 carrots diced, 3 cups vegetable broth, 1 tsp thyme, salt, pepper
- **Servings**: 4
- **Mode of cooking**: Stewing
- **Procedure**: 1. Cook onion, carrots; 2. Add lentils, tomatoes, broth, thyme, cook until lentils are tender.
- **Nutritional values**: Calories: 190, Fat: 1g, Carbs: 35g, Protein: 12g

Brown Rice Pilaf with Fresh Herbs

- **Preparation time**: 30 minutes
- **Ingredients**: 1 cup brown rice, 2 cups chicken or vegetable broth, 1/4 cup mixed fresh herbs (parsley, thyme, chives), 2 tbsp olive oil, salt, pepper
- **Servings**: 4
- **Mode of cooking**: Simmering
- **Procedure**: 1. Cook rice in broth; 2. Stir in herbs, olive oil, salt, pepper.
- **Nutritional values**: Calories: 240, Fat: 7g, Carbs: 39g, Protein: 5g

Chickpea Salad with Lemon Vinaigrette

- **Preparation time**: 15 minutes
- **Ingredients**: 1 can chickpeas drained, 1 cucumber diced, 1/2 red onion finely sliced, 1/4 cup feta cheese crumbled, 3 tbsp lemon juice, 3 tbsp olive oil, salt, pepper
- **Servings**: 4
- **Mode of cooking**: Mixing
- **Procedure**: 1. Toss chickpeas, cucumber, onion, feta; 2. Mix lemon juice, olive oil, salt, pepper, pour over salad.
- **Nutritional values**: Calories: 220, Fat: 11g, Carbs: 25g, Protein: 8g

Barley and Mushroom Risotto

- **Preparation time**: 55 minutes
- **Ingredients**: 1 cup barley, 2 cups mushrooms sliced, 1 onion diced, 4 cups vegetable broth, 1/2 cup Parmesan cheese grated, 2 tbsp olive oil, salt, pepper
- **Servings**: 4
- **Mode of cooking**: Sauteing and Simmering
- **Procedure**: 1. Saute onion, mushrooms; 2. Add barley, broth, cook until creamy; 3. Stir in Parmesan, salt, pepper.
- **Nutritional values**: Calories: 320, Fat: 12g, Carbs: 44g, Protein: 12g

Bulgur with Grilled Vegetables

- **Preparation time**: 25 minutes
- **Ingredients**: 1 cup bulgur, 2 cups mixed grilled vegetables (bell peppers, zucchini, eggplant), 3 tbsp olive oil, 1 tsp smoked paprika, salt, pepper
- **Servings**: 4
- **Method of cooking**: Boiling and Grilling
- **Procedure**: 1. Cook bulgur as per instructions; 2. Toss grilled vegetables, olive oil, paprika, salt, pepper with bulgur.

- **Nutritional values**: Calories: 220, Fat: 9g, Carbs: 31g, Protein: 6g

Black Bean and Corn Salsa

- **Preparation time**: 15 minutes
- **Ingredients**: 1 cup black beans cooked, 1 cup corn kernels, 1/2 red onion diced, 1/4 cup cilantro chopped, 2 tbsp lime juice, salt, pepper
- **Servings**: 6
- **Method of cooking**: Mixing
- **Procedure**: 1. Combine all ingredients; 2. Chill for 1 hour before serving.
- **Nutritional values**: Calories: 90, Fat: 1g, Carbs: 17g, Protein: 5g

Farro with Roasted Peppers

- **Preparation time**: 40 minutes
- **Ingredients**: 1 cup farro, 2 red bell peppers roasted and sliced, 1/4 cup feta cheese crumbled, 3 tbsp olive oil, 1 tbsp red wine vinegar, salt, pepper
- **Servings**: 4
- **Method of cooking**: Boiling and Roasting
- **Procedure**: 1. Cook farro; 2. Mix farro, peppers, feta, olive oil, vinegar, salt, pepper.

- **Nutritional values**: Calories: 250, Fat: 11g, Carbs: 33g, Protein: 7g

Spelt Berry Salad with Arugula

- **Preparation time**: 30 minutes
- **Ingredients**: 1 cup spelt berries cooked, 2 cups arugula, 1/2 cup cherry tomatoes halved, 1/4 cup shaved Parmesan, 3 tbsp balsamic vinaigrette
- **Servings**: 4
- **Method of cooking**: Mixing
- **Procedure**: 1. Toss spelt berries, arugula, tomatoes, Parmesan; 2. Drizzle with vinaigrette.
- **Nutritional values**: Calories: 180, Fat: 7g, Carbs: 24g, Protein: 6g

Millet and Vegetable Stir-Fry

- **Preparation time**: 20 minutes
- **Ingredients**: 1 cup millet cooked, 2 cups mixed vegetables (carrots, peas, bell peppers), 2 tbsp soy sauce, 1 tbsp sesame oil, 1 tsp ginger minced
- **Servings**: 4
- **Method of cooking**: Stir-frying
- **Procedure**: 1. Stir-fry vegetables in sesame oil and ginger; 2. Add millet, soy sauce; stir-fry until heated.

- **Nutritional values**: Calories: 200, Fat: 6g, Carbs: 31g, Protein: 6g

Fermented and Pickled Delights

Classic Kimchi

- **Preparation time**: 2 days (including fermentation)
- **Ingredients**: 1 head Napa cabbage, quartered and chopped, 4 tbsp sea salt, 4 cups water, 2 tbsp grated ginger, 4 minced garlic cloves, 2 tsp sugar, 3 tbsp fish sauce, 1/4 cup Korean chili flakes (gochugaru), 8 green onions chopped, 1 daikon radish julienned
- **Servings**: 10
- **Mode of cooking**: Fermentation
- **Procedure**: 1. Soak cabbage in salted water 2 hours; 2. Rinse, drain; 3. Mix ginger, garlic, sugar, fish sauce, gochugaru; 4. Combine with cabbage, onion, radish; 5. Place in jar, ferment 2 days.
- **Nutritional values**: Calories: 35, Sodium: 500mg, Carbs: 7g, Fiber: 2g

Homemade Sauerkraut

- **Preparation time**: 14 days (for fermentation)
- **Ingredients**: 2 lbs shredded green cabbage, 1 tbsp sea salt

- **Servings**: 15
- **Mode of cooking**: Fermentation
- **Procedure**: 1. Combine cabbage, salt, knead; 2. Transfer to jar, cover tightly; 3. Let ferment 2 weeks, opening periodically to release gases.
- **Nutritional values**: Calories: 20, Sodium: 400mg, Carbs: 4g, Fiber: 3g

Spicy Pickled Cucumbers

- **Preparation time**: 1 day
- **Ingredients**: 4 medium cucumbers sliced, 1 cup apple cider vinegar, 1 cup water, 2 tbsp sugar, 1 tbsp salt, 2 tsp chili flakes, 2 cloves garlic minced
- **Servings**: 8
- **Mode of cooking**: Pickling
- **Procedure**: 1. Mix vinegar, water, sugar, salt; 2. Add cucumbers, chili, garlic; 3. Refrigerate 24 hours before serving.
- **Nutritional values**: Calories: 25, Sodium: 350mg, Carbs: 6g

Fermented Beets with Dill

- **Preparation time**: 7 days
- **Ingredients**: 4 large beets peeled, sliced, 2 tbsp sea salt, 4 cups water, 3 dill sprigs
- **Servings**: 6
- **Mode of cooking**: Fermentation
- **Procedure**: 1. Dissolve salt in water; 2. Place beets, dill in jar; 3. Cover with saltwater; 4. Seal, ferment 1 week.
- **Nutritional values**: Calories: 60, Sodium: 400mg, Carbs: 13g, Fiber: 3g

Ginger Pickled Carrots

- **Preparation time**: 48 hours
- **Ingredients**: 6 large carrots julienned, 1 cup rice vinegar, 1 cup water, 1/4 cup sugar, 2 tbsp salt, 2-inch piece ginger sliced
- **Servings**: 8
- **Mode of cooking**: Pickling
- **Procedure**: 1. Boil vinegar, water, sugar, salt; 2. Add carrots, ginger; 3. Cool, store in fridge 48 hours.
- **Nutritional values**: Calories: 50, Sodium: 500mg, Carbs: 12g, Fiber: 2g

Red Cabbage Slaw with Apple Cider Vinegar

- **Preparation time**: 1 hour

- **Ingredients**: 1/2 head red cabbage shredded, 1/4 cup apple cider vinegar, 1 tbsp honey, 2 tbsp olive oil, 1/2 tsp salt, 1/4 tsp black pepper, 1 carrot shredded
- **Servings**: 4
- **Mode of cooking**: Mixing
- **Procedure**: 1. Whisk vinegar, honey, oil, salt, pepper; 2. Toss with cabbage, carrot; 3. Chill 1 hour.
- **Nutritional values**: Calories: 120, Fat: 7g, Carbs: 13g, Protein: 2g

Fermented Salsa

- **Preparation time**: 3 days
- **Ingredients**: 4 tomatoes chopped, 1 onion diced, 2 jalapeños minced, 1/4 cup cilantro chopped, 2 cloves garlic minced, 1 tsp salt, 1/4 cup whey
- **Servings**: 6
- **Mode of cooking**: Fermentation
- **Procedure**: 1. Mix all ingredients; 2. Store in jar, ferment 3 days; 3. Serve chilled.
- **Nutritional values**: Calories: 25, Sodium: 400mg, Carbs: 5g, Fiber: 1g

Pickled Red Onions

- **Preparation time**: 24 hours

- **Ingredients**: 2 red onions thinly sliced, 1 cup apple cider vinegar, 1 tbsp sugar, 1 1/2 tsp salt, 1 cup water
- **Servings**: 8
- **Mode of cooking**: Pickling
- **Procedure**: 1. Boil vinegar, water, sugar, salt; 2. Pour over onions; 3. Chill 24 hours.
- **Nutritional values**: Calories: 25, Sodium: 450mg, Carbs: 6g

Spiced Fermented Cauliflower

- **Preparation time**: 5 days
- **Ingredients**: 1 head cauliflower florets, 1 tbsp sea salt, 4 cups water, 1 tsp cumin seeds, 1 tsp coriander seeds, 2 garlic cloves
- **Servings**: 5
- **Mode of cooking**: Fermentation

- **Procedure**: 1. Dissolve salt in water; 2. Add spices, garlic to jar; 3. Add cauliflower, cover with brine; 4. Ferment 5 days.
- **Nutritional values**: Calories: 45, Sodium: 500mg, Carbs: 9g, Fiber: 4g

Probiotic Vegetable Medley

- **Preparation time**: 7 days
- **Ingredients**: 1 cup carrots sliced, 1 cup green beans, 1 red bell pepper sliced, 1 tbsp sea salt, 4 cups water, 2 bay leaves, 1 tsp black peppercorns
- **Servings**: 6
- **Mode of cooking**: Fermentation
- **Procedure**: 1. Blanch carrots, beans; 2. Layer veggies, spices in jar; 3. Cover with brine; 4. Ferment 7 days.
- **Nutritional values**: Calories: 30, Sodium: 400mg, Carbs: 7g, Fiber: 3g

Chapter 8: Fueling Hacks and Tips

Understanding Fuelings and Their Importance

In the journey of healing and wellness, the concept of 'fueling' takes on a vital role. These are not just meals or snacks; they represent a thoughtful approach to nourishing the body and mind. Understanding the philosophy behind fueling and recognizing their importance is key to transforming one's relationship with food.

The essence of fueling

At its core, a fueling is more than just a means to satiate hunger. It is about feeding your body with what it genuinely needs. This means choosing foods that not only satisfy your taste buds but also provide the necessary nutrients to energize, heal, and rejuvenate your body. For the busy entrepreneur aiming to launch a tech startup, it means selecting foods that boost cognitive function and sustain energy levels. For the mother concerned about her family's health, it's about choosing wholesome, nutrient-rich options that support her children's growth and well-being.

Fueling emphasize the consumption of whole, unprocessed foods. These are foods in their most natural state, unaltered and free from additives. Whole foods such as fruits, vegetables, whole grains, nuts, and seeds are packed with essential vitamins, minerals, antioxidants, and fibers. They are instrumental in fighting inflammation, a key factor highlighted in the first chapter of our journey.

Balancing Macronutrients

Each fueling should aim for a balance of macronutrients - carbohydrates, proteins, and fats. This balance is not just about counting calories; it's about making each calorie count.

For someone launching a startup, a balanced fueling could mean a smoothie with fruits (carbohydrates), Greek yogurt (protein), and a spoonful of almond butter (fats). For a health-conscious mother, it might be a salad with leafy greens (carbohydrates), grilled chicken (protein), and olive oil dressing (fats).

Fueling also focus on the timing and portion of meals. Eating at regular intervals can prevent overeating, manage hunger, and maintain steady energy levels throughout the day. Understanding portion sizes is crucial to avoid the common pitfall of overindulgence, even in healthy foods.

Mindful Eating

Fueling encourage mindfulness - the practice of being fully present and engaged while eating. It involves savoring each bite, listening to the body's hunger cues, and recognizing the signs of fullness. Mindful eating can transform meals from hurried necessities into moments of nourishment and reflection.

Fueling are not one-size-fits-all. They should be tailored to individual needs, preferences, and goals. For the aspiring entrepreneur, this might mean incorporating brain-boosting foods like walnuts and blueberries. For the mother, it involves selecting foods that are both nutritious and kid-friendly.

The Connection to Overall Well-being

Lastly, fueling are deeply connected to overall well-being. They are not just about physical health; they also impact mental health, energy levels, and emotional stability. A well-planned fueling strategy can lead to improved concentration, better mood, and a more balanced life.

In conclusion, fueling represent a holistic approach to eating. They are deliberate, balanced, and mindful choices that nourish the body and soul. By understanding and incorporating the concept of fueling, individuals can make significant strides in their journey towards health and wellness.

Integrating Fuelings into Your Day

In our bustling lives, whether as future tech moguls or nurturing parents, the way we fuel our bodies can profoundly impact our daily effectiveness and long-term well-being. This chapter delves into practical strategies to seamlessly integrate nutritious fueling into your daily routine.

Understanding the Role of Nutrient-Dense fueling
Fueling are more than just meals; they are the energy sources that power our ambitions and care. For an entrepreneur dreaming of launching a startup, fueling mean sustaining long hours of focus and creativity. For a mother, they involve nurturing her family with nourishing choices that foster growth and health.

The Early Morning Boost
Start your day with intention and nutrition. A robust morning routine sets the foundation for a productive day. Consider a smoothie blending leafy greens, protein-rich yogurt, and a touch of honey for an energizing start. This quick blend provides the entrepreneur the necessary brain power, while being an easy, on-the-go breakfast for busy moms.

Midday: Sustaining Your Momentum
The midday meal is pivotal. Entrepreneurs can opt for a light yet filling quinoa salad, rich in proteins and fibers, keeping them alert and focused. For mothers, a chicken and vegetable wrap, easy to prepare and appealing to children, offers a balanced midday meal.

Afternoon Snacks: Quick Energy Fixes

Afternoon slumps are common, but the right snack can make all the difference. A handful of almonds and a piece of fruit can re-energize an entrepreneur, while carrot sticks with hummus serve as a healthy snack for kids returning from school.

Evening: Unwinding and Refueling

Dinner is a time to replenish and unwind. Entrepreneurs might favor a light, protein-rich fish dish with steamed vegetables. Families can gather around a hearty vegetable stew, offering comfort and a balanced nutritional profile.

Integrating Smart Cooking Practices

Meal prepping is a game-changer. Dedicating a few hours on the weekend to prepare and store components of meals can save precious time during the week. Utilize smart cooking techniques like batch cooking, slow-cooking, and using a pressure cooker to make meal preparation efficient and hassle-free.

Listening to Your Body

Fueling is not just about what you eat but also how you eat. Mindful eating, paying attention to the body's cues of hunger and fullness, ensures that both the entrepreneur and the parent are eating for nourishment and not out of stress or distraction.

Customizing Your Fueling Plan

Tailor your fueling plan to fit your lifestyle and goals. Entrepreneurs might need more brain-boosting foods, while parents might focus on family-friendly, nutrient-rich options. Remember, there's no one-size-fits-all approach to nutrition.

The Path to Holistic Well-being

Integrating effective fueling into your day is vital for both physical health and mental clarity. Whether you're building a startup or raising a family, your diet plays a crucial role in your journey.

Embrace these tips to make nourishing food choices that align with your lifestyle and aspirations.

When and How to Use Fueling Hacks

In the fast-paced rhythm of modern life, maintaining a balance between nourishment and daily obligations can be a challenge. The art of using fueling hacks lies in their strategic implementation, ensuring that both busy professionals and active families can enjoy healthy, satisfying meals without compromising on time or quality.

Timing is Everything

1. ***Morning Kick-Start****:* For the early risers or the morning hustlers, a protein-packed smoothie can be a lifesaver. Blending a combination of Greek yogurt, fruits, and a handful of spinach offers a quick, nutrient-rich start. This approach suits the on-the-go entrepreneur and busy parents preparing for the day ahead.

2. ***Midday Recharge****:* Afternoon slumps affect everyone. A small, protein-rich snack, like a handful of nuts or a cheese stick, can provide the necessary energy boost without the heaviness of a large meal. For the working professional, this means sustained focus for afternoon tasks. For parents, it's about having the energy to match their children's after-school enthusiasm.

Smart Choices for Busy Lives

1. ***Pre-Prepared Meals****:* The modern world demands modern solutions. Preparing meals in advance or opting for healthy meal delivery services can save precious time. For those building a business or juggling family logistics, having a ready-to-eat meal that aligns with dietary goals can be a game-changer.

2. **Hydration Hacks**: Staying hydrated is key, but often overlooked. Keeping a water bottle at hand and infusing water with fruits or herbs can make hydration appealing and convenient. This simple step ensures that both the dedicated professional and the multitasking parent stay adequately hydrated throughout the day.

Fueling on the Go

1. *Portable Snacks*: Portable, healthy snacks are essential for those constantly on the move. Packing a mix of fruits, nuts, or vegetable sticks can prevent unhealthy food choices. For entrepreneurs rushing between meetings and parents running errands, these snacks provide a quick, nutritious option.
2. *Dinner Simplified*: Utilizing one-pot recipes or slow cookers can simplify dinner preparation. These methods allow for nutrient-rich meals with minimal active cooking time, ideal for a busy family or a late-working professional.

Innovative Fueling Strategies

1. *Technology to the Rescue*: Using apps for meal planning and grocery shopping can streamline the process of maintaining a healthy diet. They can suggest recipes, track nutritional intake, and even order groceries for delivery, integrating seamlessly into the digitally-driven lives of modern families and professionals.
2. *Community and Support*: Joining online communities or local groups focused on healthy eating can provide support, tips, and motivation. Sharing experiences and challenges with like-minded individuals can make the journey towards a healthier lifestyle more enjoyable and sustainable.

In conclusion, integrating fueling hacks into daily routines requires a blend of planning, smart choices, and the use of modern tools. Whether it's preparing meals in advance, choosing portable snacks, or leveraging technology, these hacks are designed to fit seamlessly into the lifestyles of those striving for health without sacrificing their ambitions or family time.

Chapter 9: Overcoming Common Challenges

Tackling Plateaus

In the realm of personal health and wellness, encountering a plateau can be both perplexing and discouraging. A plateau, often experienced during weight loss or fitness regimens, is a state where progress seems to halt despite ongoing efforts. This chapter delves into understanding and overcoming these standstills, guiding both men and women in their respective health and lifestyle goals.

Understanding the Plateau Phenomenon

A plateau is not just a barrier but a signal from your body. It indicates that your body has adapted to the current regime and requires a change to continue progressing. This understanding is vital, especially for men aiming to streamline their routines and improve dietary habits, and for women striving to balance work-life and family health.

Strategies to Overcome Plateaus

1. **Revamp Your Diet**: Sometimes, the key to pushing past a plateau lies in making dietary adjustments. Introducing more variety or altering the macronutrient balance can jumpstart the body's metabolism. For instance, incorporating more protein and fiber can enhance satiety and aid in fat loss, aligning with the goals of improving dietary habits and achieving a healthier lifestyle for the family.

2. **Intensify Your Workout**: Altering your workout intensity or type can effectively break a plateau. This could mean increasing weights, incorporating high-intensity interval training (HIIT), or trying a new form of exercise. Such changes are crucial for those looking to streamline their routines and see continuous progress.

Psychological Aspects of Plateaus

1. **Stay Motivated**: Plateaus can be mentally challenging, often leading to demotivation. Setting small, achievable goals can keep you motivated. Remember, progress is not always linear; it's about the bigger picture – maintaining a healthy lifestyle and achieving long-term wellbeing.
2. **Seek Support**: Sometimes, a fresh perspective can be beneficial. Consulting a nutritionist or a personal trainer can provide new insights and tailored strategies to overcome your specific plateau. This support is particularly valuable for individuals balancing busy work-life schedules and family responsibilities.

Innovative Approaches

1. **Track and Adjust**: Utilize apps or journals to track your diet and exercise. Monitoring progress can highlight areas needing adjustment, a tool essential for those managing a tech startup or a busy household.
2. **Rest and Recover**: Adequate rest and recovery are often underrated. Overtraining or under-recovering can lead to plateaus. Ensure you're getting enough sleep and rest days, crucial for bodily recovery and overall health.

Tackling plateaus requires a multifaceted approach, including diet and exercise adjustments, psychological strategies, and innovative tools. Understanding that plateaus are a natural part of the journey is vital. With persistence, adaptation, and the right mindset, overcoming these hurdles is not just possible but can be a stepping stone to greater achievements in your health and wellness journey.

Dietary Restrictions and Modifications

Adapting your diet to accommodate allergies, sensitivities, or health conditions is a proactive journey towards wellness. It's about making informed choices, like substituting nuts with seeds or choosing gluten-free grains. These adjustments ensure that your meals are safe, nutritious, and enjoyable, aligning with your goal of improving dietary habits without sacrificing pleasure.

Ethical and Environmental Choices

For those guided by ethical or environmental concerns, embracing plant-based alternatives is more than a diet change; it's a lifestyle choice. Swapping animal products for plant-based options like legumes and tofu not only aligns with ethical values but also enriches your diet with essential nutrients. This approach is especially relevant for maintaining a balanced family lifestyle, ensuring that your dietary choices are both healthful and principled.

Navigating dietary restrictions is as much about educating yourself as it is about informing others. Understanding the nuances of your dietary needs and effectively communicating them ensures that your lifestyle, whether busy with entrepreneurial endeavors or family care, is not hindered by dietary limitations. Supplementing your diet and meal prepping are part of an integrative approach that accommodates your health needs while fitting seamlessly into your daily routine.

In conclusion, managing dietary restrictions and modifications is a journey of balance and understanding, where each choice is a step towards a healthier and more harmonious lifestyle. Whether it's for health, ethical, or environmental reasons, these dietary adjustments are a testament to your commitment to wellbeing.

Managing Social and Dining Out Situations

Dining out presents a unique set of challenges for those committed to a Lean and Green lifestyle. It's about finding harmony between social enjoyment and dietary goals. Start by researching restaurants in advance, focusing on those offering fresh, whole foods. Once there, don't hesitate to engage with the staff about menu modifications that align with your dietary needs. Opt for grilled over fried items, request dressings and sauces on the side, and prioritize lean proteins and greens. This strategy not only aligns with your goal to streamline daily routines but also ensures that your dining out experience supports your health objectives.

Social Settings: Balancing Enjoyment and Health Goals

In social situations, particularly those revolving around food, striking a balance is key. When attending gatherings or parties, consider eating a nutritious meal beforehand to avoid overindulgence. Alternatively, offering to bring a Lean and Green dish not only ensures there's something you can enjoy but also introduces others to your healthy lifestyle. This approach resonates particularly with those striving to maintain a work-life balance and instill healthy habits within their family.

Effective communication is vital in managing social and dining out situations. Don't shy away from discussing your dietary preferences with friends, family, and restaurant staff. Advocating for your health needs is a demonstration of self-care and commitment to your wellbeing.

This proactive stance is especially relevant for individuals juggling the demands of a tech startup or managing a busy family life. It ensures that your dietary choices are respected and accommodated, thus preventing any discomfort or misunderstanding.

In essence, managing social and dining out situations on a Lean and Green diet is about preparation, communication, and balance. It's about making informed choices that align with your health goals while enjoying the social aspects of dining. With these strategies, you can confidently navigate any social situation, ensuring that your dietary habits support both your personal and professional aspirations.

Chapter 10: Drink Right, Stay Hydrated

Herbal Teas and Their Benefits

In a world where health and wellness are paramount, herbal teas emerge as a key player. These teas, steeped in tradition and nature's goodness, offer more than just hydration—they are a portal to holistic well-being. This section explores the multifaceted benefits of herbal teas and their seamless integration into a healthy lifestyle.

The Essence of Herbal Teas

Herbal teas, or tisanes, are not just beverages but a blend of nature's finest herbs, spices, and botanicals. Each variety brings its own unique health benefits and flavors. For instance, chamomile is celebrated for its calming properties, aiding in relaxation and sleep, while peppermint tea is a go-to for digestive health. The caffeine-free nature of these teas makes them a perfect choice for all-day enjoyment, aligning with the goals of a Lean and Green lifestyle.

Daily Integration and Benefits

Incorporating herbal teas into daily life is both enjoyable and beneficial. Starting the day with invigorating green tea or a cup of lemon balm can energize and refresh. Midday, when stress might peak, options like lavender or hibiscus provide a soothing escape. Evening brings an opportunity for rest and relaxation, where teas like valerian or passionflower promote peaceful sleep. For those managing dietary restrictions, the wide array of herbal teas offers a versatile, healthful, and inclusive beverage choice.

Beyond Hydration: A Lifestyle Choice

Herbal teas are more than a hydration choice; they are a lifestyle decision. Each sip is an exploration into the realm of natural healing, offering a moment to pause and connect with the environment. They fit perfectly into the Lean and Green ethos, providing health benefits, satisfying cravings without calories, and supporting overall well-being. Embracing herbal teas is about nurturing the body, calming the mind, and indulging in the richness of flavors nature has to offer.

In embracing herbal teas, one not only chooses a healthier hydration option but also steps into a world of natural wellness, uncovering the harmonious balance between human health and the botanical world.

Delicious and Nutritious Smoothies

In the landscape of health and vitality, smoothies stand out as a versatile and delightful way to nourish the body. This chapter explores the art of creating delicious and nutritious smoothies, perfectly aligning with the Lean and Green lifestyle's commitment to health and wellness.

The Power of Smoothies

Smoothies are more than just a blend of ingredients; they are a symphony of flavors and nutrients, offering a convenient and delicious way to consume a variety of fruits, vegetables, and proteins.

For busy professionals and health-conscious families alike, smoothies provide a quick, nutrient-packed meal option that can be tailored to individual tastes and dietary needs. They are an excellent way to ensure intake of essential vitamins, minerals, and antioxidants, supporting overall health and well-being.

Crafting the Perfect Smoothie

The key to a great smoothie lies in its composition. A balance of leafy greens, ripe fruits, lean proteins, and healthy fats creates a nutritious and satisfying drink. Ingredients like spinach, kale, and avocado bring in the green goodness, while fruits like berries, bananas, and mangoes add natural sweetness and fiber. For an added protein boost, incorporating Greek yogurt, nut butters, or plant-based protein powders can transform a smoothie into a fulfilling meal. These ingredients not only enhance the smoothie's nutritional profile but also provide sustained energy, making them ideal for breakfast, post-workout recovery, or a midday snack.

Personalizing Your Smoothie

One of the greatest strengths of smoothies is their adaptability. Whether catering to dietary restrictions, managing weight, or simply seeking variety, smoothies can be customized to fit any need. For those on a low-carb diet, focusing on high-fiber, low-sugar fruits and adding healthy fats like chia seeds or coconut oil can maintain the balance. For individuals with specific health goals, such as boosting immunity or enhancing digestion, adding superfoods like spirulina, turmeric, or ginger can provide targeted benefits. The possibilities are endless, allowing for creativity and personal preference to lead the way.

In embracing the world of smoothies, individuals embark on a journey of flavor and nutrition, discovering new ways to enjoy the abundance of nature's bounty. Smoothies are not just a drink; they are a lifestyle choice that encourages health, convenience, and the joy of eating well.

Hydration Hacks and Why Water is Key

In a world bustling with myriad beverage options, the simple act of drinking water still reigns supreme in maintaining health and vitality. This chapter delves into why water is indispensable for our bodies and offers practical tips to stay effectively hydrated.

The Essence of Hydration

Water is the foundation of life. It's not just about quenching thirst; it's about nurturing every cell in our bodies. For the active professional, the busy parent, or anyone aiming for a healthier lifestyle, understanding the role of water is pivotal. It regulates body temperature, aids digestion, flushes out toxins, and even helps in weight management. In the context of a Lean and Green lifestyle, where optimal nutrition is key, water plays a vital role in enhancing the benefits of a balanced diet.

Making Hydration a Habit

Integrating adequate water intake into daily life can be challenging, but it's not insurmountable. One effective approach is to start the day with a glass of water. This simple act kick-starts metabolism and signals the body to begin its daily functions. Incorporating water-rich foods like cucumbers, zucchini, and watermelon into meals is another excellent way to boost hydration. For those who find plain water monotonous, adding a splash of lemon, cucumber slices, or a few berries can enhance the flavor, making it more appealing.

Tracking and Reminders

In today's digital age, leveraging technology can be a game-changer in maintaining hydration levels. Numerous apps are available that remind you to drink water at regular intervals. Even setting simple alarms can be effective. For those who prefer a more traditional approach, carrying a refillable water bottle serves as a constant physical reminder. The goal is to make water intake a conscious and consistent part of the daily routine.

Hydration for Active Lifestyles

For individuals with active lifestyles or those who engage in regular workouts, staying hydrated is even more crucial. Water supports muscle function and helps prevent fatigue and cramps. During extended activities, sipping water at regular intervals can provide sustained energy. Post-exercise, water aids in recovery and helps the body rebuild.

In essence, while exploring the vast landscape of nutrition and wellness, water remains a constant ally. It's about more than just staying hydrated; it's about embracing a lifestyle where water is as integral as the food we eat. This chapter aims not just to inform but to transform the way we view and consume water – making it a deliberate and enjoyable part of our health journey.

Chapter 11: The Vegan and Vegetarian Lean and Green Way

Adapting the Lean and Green Approach

Embracing a plant-based lifestyle within the Lean and Green framework is not just about removing animal products; it's about creatively incorporating a rich variety of plant-based proteins, nutrients, and flavors into your diet.

Plant-Based Protein Power

Transitioning to a plant-based Lean and Green diet calls for a focus on protein-rich foods like legumes, tofu, and quinoa. These ingredients not only supplement your protein needs but also offer a spectrum of nutrients crucial for overall health. Understanding the art of combining these proteins to form complete amino acid profiles is key. This shift also encourages exploring diverse food sources, ensuring a well-rounded intake of essential nutrients often missed in traditional diets.

Culinary Creativity and Mindful Planning

Adopting a vegetarian or vegan Lean and Green approach opens avenues for culinary creativity. Experiment with an array of herbs and spices, and explore international vegan and vegetarian cuisines. Staples like spinach and tofu stir-fry or lentil shepherd's pie can transform your meals into nutritious, flavor-packed experiences. Equally important is mindful meal planning. Structured weekly meal plans, strategic grocery shopping, and batch cooking can keep you aligned with your health goals while offering diverse and satisfying meal options.

In summary, adapting to a vegan or vegetarian Lean and Green diet is a journey of exploration and creativity. It's an opportunity to connect with a wide range of ingredients and cuisines while ensuring your meals are balanced and nutritious. With a bit of planning and a willingness to try new things, you can enjoy a diverse, fulfilling plant-based diet that aligns with the Lean and Green principles.

Protein Sources for Plant-Based Diets

Navigating the world of plant-based nutrition can often lead to the crucial question: "Where do I get my protein?" This section delves into the variety of protein sources available in a vegan and vegetarian diet, breaking the myth that adequate protein intake is only possible through animal products.

Diverse Sources of Plant-Based Protein

The cornerstone of plant-based protein lies in understanding the variety available. Legumes like lentils, chickpeas, and black beans are not only high in protein but also rich in fiber and other nutrients. Tofu, tempeh, and seitan offer versatility and can be used in a myriad of recipes, from stir-fries to grills. Quinoa and amaranth, ancient grains, provide a complete protein profile, while nuts and seeds like almonds, chia, and hemp seeds add not only protein but also essential omega-3 fatty acids to your diet.

Integrating Protein into Meals

It's important to strategically integrate these protein sources into daily meals. Start your day with a chia seed and banana smoothie, incorporate a quinoa salad for lunch, and end with a hearty lentil stew for dinner.

Snacking on hummus with vegetables or a handful of almonds can keep your protein levels topped up throughout the day. The goal is to spread protein intake evenly, ensuring a constant supply for the body's needs.

Beyond the Protein - A Holistic Approach

Embracing a plant-based diet is more than just focusing on protein. It's about creating a balanced and varied dietary pattern that includes a wide spectrum of vitamins, minerals, and other essential nutrients. Regularly including a colorful array of fruits and vegetables ensures a comprehensive nutrient intake, fostering overall health and well-being.

In conclusion, adopting a vegan or vegetarian diet within the Lean and Green framework offers a plethora of protein-rich options. By exploring and integrating a diverse range of plant-based proteins into your daily meals, you can enjoy a nutritious, balanced, and exciting dietary journey. Remember, the key is variety and balance, ensuring that your body receives all the essential nutrients it needs to thrive.

Delicious Plant-Based Recipes

Plant-Powered Mornings

Kickstart your day with vibrant, nourishing breakfasts. Imagine a warm bowl of oatmeal, rich with fresh berries and flax seeds, sweetened with a dash of agave. Or blend up a revitalizing smoothie combining spinach, banana, almond milk, and a scoop of pea protein for those busy mornings. These breakfasts are not only energizing but also a delightful way to wake up your taste buds.

Energizing Lunches and Dinners

Lunches that keep you fueled and dinners that satisfy are key in a plant-based diet. For a fulfilling midday meal, try a chickpea salad sandwich, blending mashed chickpeas with vegan mayo and a hint of dill. Or opt for a colorful quinoa and black bean bowl, adorned with avocado and cherry tomatoes. As the day winds down, enjoy a hearty lentil shepherd's pie topped with creamy mashed potatoes or a light, flavorful tofu stir-fry with mixed vegetables in a soy-ginger sauce.

Snacks, Sides, and Sweet Indulgences

Snack time offers endless possibilities like roasted spiced chickpeas or crisp cucumber slices with homemade hummus. Elevate your meals with sides like balsamic-glazed Brussels sprouts or a refreshing kale and lemon-tahini salad. And for dessert, treat yourself to a mango-topped chia pudding or homemade vegan dark chocolate and almond butter cups, proving that plant-based eating can be both healthy and decadently delicious.

In this chapter, we explore how a plant-based diet can be diverse, flavorsome, and satisfying. These recipes cater to various tastes and preferences, proving that vegan and vegetarian diets are far from monotonous. Whether you're fully committed to plant-based eating or just incorporating more veggie-centric meals into your diet, these recipes offer healthful, delicious options for every meal of the day.

Appendices

1. ***Measurement Conversions***

   Navigating through diverse recipes often means encountering various units of measurement. This section is an invaluable tool, making the transition between grams and ounces or liters and cups seamless. It's designed to ensure accuracy in your cooking, helping you maintain consistency in flavor and nutrition, irrespective of the measuring standards used in the recipe.

2. ***Glossary of Terms***

   Embarking on a vegan or vegetarian journey introduces a plethora of new ingredients and cooking techniques. The glossary serves as your culinary compass, explaining terms like 'tempeh', 'seitan', or 'aquafaba'. This knowledge enriches your cooking experience, demystifying the world of plant-based cuisine.

3. ***Recommended Reading and Resources***

   Continued learning is key to maintaining and enhancing a vegan or vegetarian lifestyle. This section offers a curated list of books, websites, and online forums that provide insights into plant-based nutrition, innovative recipes, and tips for sustainable living. These resources are selected to inspire and guide you through every step of your journey.

4. ***Acknowledgements and About the Author***

   This space is dedicated to expressing gratitude to those who contributed to the creation of this guide. It also provides a brief insight into the author's journey and expertise in plant-based cooking, lending a personal touch and establishing a connection with the reader.

In conclusion, the appendices of this chapter are not just afterthoughts but essential components that complement the main content. They are designed to empower you, enrich your understanding, and provide practical tools to navigate the vegan or vegetarian lifestyle with confidence and ease.

Measurement Conversions

Volume Equivalents (Liquid)

US Standard	US Standard (ounces)	Metric (approximate)
2 tablespoons	1 fl. oz.	30 mL
¼ cup	2 fl. oz.	60 mL
half cup	4 fl. oz.	120 mL
1 cup	8 fl. oz.	240 mL
1 half cups	12 fl. oz.	355 mL
2 cups or 1 pint	16 fl. oz.	457 mL
4 cups or 1 quart	32 fl. oz.	1 L
1 gallon	128 fl. oz.	4 L

Volume Equivalents (Dry)

US Standard	Metric (approximate)
1/8 teaspoon	0.5 mL
¼ teaspoon	1 mL
half teaspoon	2 mL
¾ teaspoon	4 mL
1 teaspoon	5 mL
1 tablespoon	15 mL

¼ cup	59 mL
1/3 cup	79 mL
half cup	118 mL
2/3 cup	156 mL
¾ cup	177 mL
1 cup	235 mL
2 cups or 1 pint	475 mL
3 cups	700 mL
4 cups or 1 quart	1 L

Oven Temperatures

Fahrenheit (F)	Celsius (C) (approximate)
250°F	120°C
300°F	150°C
325°F	165°C
350°F	180°C
375°F	190°C
400°F	200°C
425°F	220°C
450°F	230°C

Weight Equivalents

US Standard	Metric (approximate)
1 tablespoon	15 g
half ounce	15 g
1 ounce	30 g

2 ounces	60 g
4 ounces	115 g
8 ounces	225 g
12 ounces	340 g
16 ounces or 1 pound or 1 lb	455 g

Glossary of Terms

In the journey of adopting a vegan or vegetarian lifestyle, you'll encounter a plethora of unique terms and ingredients that may be new and unfamiliar. This glossary serves as a comprehensive guide to understanding these terms, ensuring that your culinary adventure is both educational and enjoyable.

1. Plant-Based Proteins:

Understanding various sources of plant-based proteins is crucial for a balanced diet. This section explains terms like 'Tofu', 'Seitan', 'Tempeh', and 'Lentils', detailing their nutritional values and how they can be creatively incorporated into your meals.

2. Dairy Alternatives:

Dairy alternatives are essential in vegan diets. This part of the glossary delves into options such as 'Almond Milk', 'Soy Milk', 'Cashew Cheese', and 'Coconut Yogurt', providing insights into their uses and benefits.

3. Grains and Legumes:

Grains and legumes form the backbone of many vegetarian dishes. Learn about different types like 'Quinoa', 'Amaranth', 'Chickpeas', and 'Black Beans', including tips on preparation and health benefits.

4. Superfoods:

This section highlights nutrient-rich superfoods like 'Chia Seeds', 'Flaxseeds', 'Kale', and 'Acai Berries'. Discover why these foods are labeled as 'super' and how to incorporate them into your diet.

5. Cooking Techniques:

Familiarize yourself with various cooking techniques that are particularly useful in plant-based cooking, such as 'Blanching', 'Steaming', 'Sautéing', and 'Marinating'. These terms will help you understand recipes better and enhance your cooking skills.

6. Flavor Enhancers:

Explore a variety of natural flavor enhancers that can elevate your dishes. Terms like 'Nutritional Yeast', 'Tamari', 'Miso', and 'Tahini' are explained, giving you insights into their use for adding depth and richness to your meals.

7. Health and Nutrition Terms:

This part covers important health and nutrition terms like 'Complete Proteins', 'Omega-3 Fatty Acids', 'Probiotics', and 'Antioxidants'. Understanding these terms is key to maintaining a healthy and well-balanced vegan or vegetarian diet.

8. Miscellaneous Terms:

Finally, this section covers additional terms that you may come across, such as 'Agar-Agar' (a gelatin substitute), 'Arrowroot Powder' (a thickening agent), and 'Aquafaba' (chickpea brine used as an egg substitute).

By providing clear and concise definitions, the glossary equips you with the knowledge to confidently navigate through recipes and make informed choices about the ingredients you use. It's an indispensable tool in your journey towards a healthful and sustainable vegan or vegetarian lifestyle.

Recommended Reading and Resources

In the pursuit of a well-informed and enriching vegan or vegetarian journey, the right resources can be transformative. This section is dedicated to providing a curated list of readings and resources that will enrich your understanding, provide practical tips, and inspire your culinary explorations.

1. Essential Literature for Plant-Based Diets:

Discover seminal works that have shaped the understanding of plant-based nutrition. Titles include:

- "How Not to Die" by Dr. Michael Greger - A comprehensive guide exploring how a plant-based diet can prevent and reverse various diseases.
- "The China Study" by T. Colin Campbell and Thomas M. Campbell II - A groundbreaking study linking the consumption of animal products with chronic illnesses.
- "Eat to Live" by Dr. Joel Fuhrman - This book focuses on nutrient-dense, plant-rich eating and its benefits for weight loss and health.

2. Cookbooks for Creative Cooking:

Explore a range of cookbooks that offer creative and delicious recipes for every occasion. Some top picks are:

- "Oh She Glows" by Angela Liddon - A collection of vegan recipes that are perfect for anyone wanting to experiment with plant-based meals.
- "Thug Kitchen: Eat Like You Give a F*ck" - A no-nonsense approach to cooking hearty, plant-based meals.
- "Veganomicon" by Isa Chandra Moskowitz and Terry Hope Romero - Known as the ultimate vegan cookbook, it covers everything from basics to advanced recipes.

3. Online Resources and Blogs:

Stay updated with the latest in plant-based eating through various online platforms. Recommended are:

- NutritionFacts.org - Dr. Michael Greger's site providing the latest in nutrition research.
- Minimalist Baker - A blog offering simple and delicious vegan recipes, most of which require 10 ingredients or less.
- Vegan Richa - A blog specializing in easy and flavorful vegan recipes with an emphasis on Indian cuisine.

4. Documentaries and Films:

Visual resources can be powerful. Include in your watchlist:

- "Forks Over Knives" - Examines the profound claim that most chronic diseases can be controlled by rejecting animal-based and processed foods.
- "Game Changers" - This documentary explores the impact of plant-based eating on physical performance and health.
- "What the Health" - Investigates the link between diet and disease, and the billions of dollars at stake in the healthcare, pharmaceutical, and food industries.

5. Apps and Digital Tools:

Leverage technology to support your diet with apps such as:

- HappyCow - An invaluable resource for finding vegan and vegetarian restaurants worldwide.
- MyFitnessPal - Useful for tracking nutrition and ensuring a balanced plant-based diet.
- Cronometer - Offers detailed nutrition tracking and is particularly helpful for monitoring micronutrient intake.

By delving into these resources, you gain not just knowledge, but also a community and a wealth of inspiration. Each book, blog, documentary, and app can be a stepping stone in your journey towards a healthier, more sustainable lifestyle that aligns with your vegan or vegetarian values.

Acknowledgements About the Author

Journey to a Plant-Based Philosophy:

Tessa Maddox's story isn't just about food; it's a narrative of transformation and commitment.

From her early days, learning the importance of fresh, garden-sourced ingredients, Tessa was destined to advocate for a healthier, more sustainable way of life. Her education at the Culinary Institute of America and subsequent diverse culinary experiences have been integral to her journey towards embracing and promoting a plant-based diet.

A Personal and Professional Odyssey:

Tessa's transition to veganism was a personal choice fueled by health and ethical considerations, marking a pivotal chapter in her life. Professionally, she has worn many hats – from a chef in acclaimed kitchens to a consultant for health-focused ventures. Her approach is deeply rooted in the belief that our food choices are powerful tools for positive change, impacting not just our health but the world around us.

Gratitude and Collaborations:

In penning this book, Tessa extends heartfelt thanks to those who have been instrumental in her journey. She acknowledges her mentor, Chef Julianne Moore, for being a guiding light, and expresses appreciation for the vibrant community of farmers, artisans, and fellow chefs who have enriched her understanding and appreciation of plant-based cuisine.

Forward-Looking and Inspirational:

As Tessa Maddox looks towards the future, her focus remains steadfast on advocating for plant-based living that's both enjoyable and sustainable. Through her book, she seeks to inspire a wider audience, advocating for a world where our dietary choices resonate with our values for health, compassion, and environmental stewardship.

Tessa's Vision:

At the heart of Tessa's work is a vision that transcends the kitchen. It's about nurturing a global community where mindful eating becomes a cornerstone of a healthier, more compassionate world.

Her culinary expertise, combined with her advocacy, paves the way for a future where plant-based living is not just a dietary choice, but a path to holistic well-being.

Made in the USA
Columbia, SC
18 December 2024

49816616R00059